SO-AKU-142

THE RECLAIM DIET

A Four-Step, Real-Food Plan For Weight Loss And Vibrant Health

ERIN CHAMERLIK, MS

Copyright © 2020
WHITE HAT FREE PRESS
ERIN CHAMERLIK, MS
THE RECLAIM DIET
A Four-Step, Real-Food Plan For Weight Loss And Vibrant Health
All rights reserved.

No part of this publication may be reproduced, distributed, or transmitted in any form or by any means, including photocopying, recording, or other electronic or mechanical methods, without the prior written permission of the publisher, except in the case of brief quotations embodied in critical reviews and certain other non-commercial uses permitted by copyright law.

WHITE HAT FREE PRESS
ERIN CHAMERLIK, MS

Printed in the United States of America
First Printing 2020
First Edition 2020

10 9 8 7 6 5 4 3 2 1

This book is not intended as a substitute for any advice, medical care and/or treatment of the reader's physician. If you suspect that you have a medical problem, please seek competent medical help. The reader should not stop prescription medications without the advice and guidance of his or her personal physician. All matters regarding your health require medical supervision. The author shall not be liable or responsible for any loss or damage allegedly arising from any information or suggestion in this book.

Names and characteristics of some of the clients portrayed in this book may have been changed. Mention of specific companies, organizations, or authorities in this book does not imply endorsement by the author. Internet addresses given in this book were accurate at the time it went to press. The author assumes no responsibility for errors, or for changes that occur after publication. Further, the author does not have any control over and does not assume any responsibility for author or third-party websites or their content.

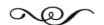

This book is dedicated to Bill, Carly and Paige

— my family, my supporters, my treasures.

TABLE OF CONTENTS

PART I

Start Here

Have You Been Duped By the Wrong Advice? Reclaim your life!

CHAPTER 1

DO YOU FEEL LIKE YOUR HEALTH IS SPINNING OUT OF CONTROL?

WELCOME! RECLAIMING HEALTH NATURALLY BEGINS WITH A CHOICE.

Congratulations! You have decided to move forward and take action to restore your health naturally. You are going to learn the simple truths about why we are sick and what to do about it. This book will guide you through a plan that works.

It has worked for me. It has worked for others, and it will work for you!

I have been helping people fix their health naturally for about 18 years.

- I fixed my own health naturally when modern medicine failed to help me with panic attacks and chronic hives.
- I fixed my blood sugar problems when the Standard American Diet led me into diabetes.
- I fixed my hormonal imbalance after synthetic birth control pills left me in a hormonal mess with Hashimoto's hypothyroidism.

I am grateful that my health journey and desire to learn all I could about natural health and wellness led me to study holistic nutrition and earn the degree of *Master of Science in Health and Nutrition Education.*

From health challenges to health victories

I needed this book two decades ago when my symptoms began appearing. I was not a nutritionist back then. I didn't eat all that well, and I did what most people do—I went to the doctor for help. When my doctor suggested that I start on antidepressant medication to cure my hives, I knew I needed to find my own answers.

I spent time with many doctors, including an allergist and internal medicine physician. The doctors offered me nothing more than prescription medications, but my condition did not improve.

I had a few other health challenges that led me to find answers through real food and natural solutions. I used my knowledge of medicine and science to research the field of nutrition, developing programs and educational materials to help individuals learn how to incorporate simple strategies to improve health and wellness.

After healing myself, it fueled my passion to help as many people as possible. Eighteen years later, and I am thrilled to have the opportunity to help people reclaim their health and their lives!

One such person was Melissa, who faced extreme pain and weight fluctuations after giving birth to her first child.

"I started to see the weight melt off."

Melissa began to experience extreme fatigue and pain after the birth of her first child. Her hands hurt so much that she was unable to dress her baby. She went to the doctor and was tested for arthritis and other ailments, but they came up negative.

"The doctor didn't know what was wrong with me, so he prescribed antidepressant medication," Melissa shared.

A few years later, her face started turning red and swollen and her skin was flaky. She was diagnosed with acne rosacea and told there was nothing she could do to prevent the condition from getting worse. Melissa was overweight and had tried many diets along the way, including Weight Watchers and Jenny Craig.

"Everything worked for a little while, but eventually I would end up putting the weight back on."

Melissa joined one of my coaching groups and learned how to eat meals and snacks based on whole, unprocessed foods. She ate an anti-inflammatory diet, removing gluten, dairy and processed food.

"I started to see the weight melt off. I noticed that the pain and fatigue improved as I stayed on the eating plan. My face looked like it had years before all the trouble began! No more puffy, red face and I lost a total of 26 pounds, and aches and pains are gone!" — Melissa Filippi

CHAPTER 2

ARE HURRIED DOCTORS MISSING THE ELEPHANT IN THE ROOM??

Check all that apply.

Are you:
- ✓ Sick or suffering
- ✓ Fat or frustrated
- ✓ Tired or wired
- ✓ Moody or medicated
- ✓ Despondent or depressed
- ✓ Anxious or agitated
- ✓ Pained and inflamed
- ✓ Sugar or grain addicted

For everything you checked, the question is, why?

"Why?" is a powerful question. Unfortunately the mainstream medical system does not ask that question. When you present yourself to a doctor you are given a few minutes to describe your symptoms. Most doctors work in the broken model that is not healthcare, rather it is SICKcare. Physicians are not compensated to spend time trying to find the *"why"* behind your symptoms. And, it is not unusual for primary care physicians to have patient appointments scheduled every 15 minutes.

In addition to being hurried in patient appointments, doctors are not trained in medical school to understand that finding and fixing the root cause can eliminate the need for medication and even surgery.

"Today, most medical schools in the United States teach less than 25 hours of nutrition over four years. The fact that less than 20% of medical schools have a single required course in nutrition—it's a scandal. It's outrageous. It's obscene." — Dr. David Eisenberg, Harvard T.H. Chan School of Public Health (1)

We need to understand that physicians are trained to prescribe but most are not trained to figure out why you are sick. The pharmaceutical industry, driven by capitalism, spends $6 billion each year marketing directly to you with commercials and advertisements. The industry spends $20 billion to influence medical students and physicians, according to an analysis published in *JAMA*, 2019 (2).

If pharmaceutical drugs solved problems and made people well without side effects, we would all be healthier after taking medication. We are not healthier. Clearly, as a nation, we are sick!

When people visit their doctor and present with high blood sugar, high blood pressure and high cholesterol, they might be given three prescriptions by their physician during a 15-minute appointment. If physicians were better trained in medical school about nutrition and lifestyle options, and if they were compensated to take time working on the underlying problem—poor diet and inactivity—patients would have better outcomes.

There are physicians across America who do understand the power of nutrition and they are teaching patients about the benefits of eating a healthy diet. Some are even promoting nutrition and cooking classes. There are conferences bringing together hundreds of physicians for the purpose of nutrition education. Teaching kitchens are springing up across the country, in hospitals and other medical facilities, teaching people how to make healthy choices and how to prepare real, unprocessed food. Sadly, this is not the norm in this country.

While we are hopeful that someday doctors will have the time and knowledge to begin the conversation about nutrition with patients, we cannot wait. I encourage you to begin the nutrition conversation with your doctor, an important member of your team. Your physician will be able to evaluate your medications and can guide you through decreasing or discontinuing medications as you make changes in your diet.

You and your doctor may be missing a huge red flag

In a way, physicians today are like investigators grabbing clues, trying to quickly figure out which drugs to prescribe. All the while they are missing the elephant in the room—the patient, the person with chronically high insulin levels.

Everyone hears the obesity statistics—93 million Americans are obese—that's enough people to fill a football stadium holding 100,000 people, every single day for two and a half years, with just obese people. While physicians may suspect that an obese person is running toward heart disease, diabetes, degenerative joint disease and cancer, they are missing the root cause in these people and they are missing the same root cause in patients of all sizes, including normal weight and under weight.

Overweight people are not lazy and unwilling to comply with weight loss advice, as many medical professionals and normal weight people believe. They are not getting diabetes because they are fat. It is estimated that 20% of overweight people are metabolically healthy but there are plenty of normal weight and thin people who aren't metabolically healthy, and at a higher risk for disease. We are judging overweight and obese people and repeating the same wrong message, "Just eat less and exercise more." More and more researchers and physicians are realizing that the exploding rates of diabetes and obesity can no longer be explained away by the flawed calorie theory—"a calorie is a calorie." We will dive deeper into this theory in Part 2.

Type 2 diabetes is one of the first obvious health dominos to fall. The problem is, by the time people are diagnosed with prediabetes or diabetes, the horse is out of the barn. Without understanding what causes the diabetes domino to fall, this disease can lead to a series of other health dominos falling.

Diabetes is connected to other diseases, including heart disease, dementia and cancer. The *British Journal of Cancer* published a report that shows the higher your average blood sugar, the higher your risk of developing cancer (3). David Perlmutter, MD, explained in his book, *Grain Brain*, that having an elevated blood sugar level increases your risk of developing many health problems. "Like a shard of glass, the toxic sugar inflicts a lot of damage, leading to blindness, infections, nerve damage, heart disease, and, yes, Alzheimer's (p. 29)."

The domino never has to fall. If you are reading this book, it is very likely that you have diabetes or prediabetes and don't even know it. You may be overweight or underweight, but if you are eating the typical American diet, you are headed for trouble. Instead of blaming overweight and obese people for being fat, we can blame those who played a part in convincing Americans that we need to follow the government dietary guidelines. We can blame government food subsidies that lead to cheap, highly refined, mass-produced food containing wheat, corn and soy. We can blame the food industry for putting inflammatory soybean oil, high in linoleic acid, in processed food. Excessive amounts of linoleic acid are strongly linked to insulin resistance, diabetes and obesity (4). Consumption of cheap soybean oil, nonexistent in the food supply in 1900, increased >1000-fold from 1909 to 1999 (5).

The CDC reported that more than 114 million U.S. adults—a staggering 44%— are living with diabetes or prediabetes, yet 31% are unaware that they have diagnosable diabetes or prediabetes. The changes that lead to diabetes begin to happen in your body years before your doctor will notice that your blood sugar levels are abnormal. You might not have any symptoms in the early stages, but the damage is accumulating in your body. The biggest change that happens silently, at first, is chronically high insulin levels. Insulin is the hormone that regulates blood sugar in the body. When everything is working smoothly, the carbohydrate food you eat is broken down into blood sugar, glucose. Insulin helps glucose enter cells where it is used for energy. Sometimes people have a history of eating carbohydrates and sugar all day long in the form of cereal with fruit and milk, or bagels and juice for breakfast, a mid-morning granola bar, a fast food burger, fries and soda at lunch, spaghetti, corn and bread at dinner, popcorn after dinner and an ice cream treat before bed. That is how I ate for years, and my diet aligned pretty well with the 1992 food pyramid. I was a thin person with insulin resistance, and nobody knew I was metabolically unhealthy. The elephant in the room is chronically high insulin levels caused by eating large amounts of processed and refined foods that are full of harmful ingredients and too many carbohydrates, keeping us food addicted.

The standard American diet tends to include a lot of highly processed foods that trick your taste buds and fool your brain into thinking that you are not satisfied. The food industry knows how to create packaged food with just the right combination of cheap oils, refined grains, artificial flavors and sugar to keep you addicted and coming back for more. Our modern diet is largely to blame for insulin resistance and associated problems with weight gain and type 2 diabetes. This addictive, damaging way of eating, coupled with modern day stress and sleep problems, comes together to create the metabolic mess we have in this country.

Your blood sugar tests (fasting glucose and Hemoglobin A1C) may appear normal because glucose is being kept in check by ever-increasing amounts of insulin. Living with high insulin levels damages health in countless ways, yet doctors are not testing insulin levels as an annual screen. High insulin levels can make you feel hungry all the time, and crave starchy and sugary foods.

When doctors focus only on monitoring our fasting glucose levels and hemoglobin A1C (a test that indicates your average blood sugar levels over the past three months), this delays identifying the root cause, chronically high insulin, for several years, even decades. By testing only your fasting glucose and hemoglobin A1C at your annual physical exam, you may be misled to believe that there are no problems to address. An important question to ask is, "Do I have chronically high insulin (hyperinsulinemia)?" Our doctors should be measuring the fasting insulin level along with fasting glucose and possibly doing further tests to see how our insulin levels respond when we are given carbohydrates (oral glucose tolerance test with insulin levels).

Signs of chronically high insulin (6, 7)

- Belly fat and an expanding waistline
- Elevated blood pressure
- Swollen ankles and fluid accumulating anywhere in your body
- High blood triglycerides
- Skin tags

- Areas of dark skin or discoloration in the creases of the neck and body folds, especially armpits, groin and neck
- Women, polycystic ovarian syndrome or gestational diabetes
- Men, low testosterone, erectile dysfunction
- Family members with type 2 diabetes
- Gout

It is very complicated to understand the hormone insulin. Every system in the body is affected by high insulin levels. Many of our modern diseases are less about genetics and more about improper diet, inadequate sleep, runaway stress and inactivity. What is the common thread among conditions like type 2 diabetes, Alzheimer's disease, acne, gout, erectile dysfunction, polycystic ovarian syndrome and mysterious conditions like vertigo and tinnitus? Researchers Fung and Berger stated, "A growing body of evidence suggests that these wide-ranging and seemingly unconnected conditions can, in fact, be linked to a common underlying cause: metabolic derangement resulting primarily from chronic hyperinsulinemia, and its eventual end point, insulin resistance (8)."

If you have any of the symptoms listed above, the good news is that you can absolutely take action now and stop the progression of declining health and accumulating fat. Chronically high insulin levels and type 2 diabetes can be avoided and often reversed and you can absolutely return to good health. The information that you will learn in this book will guide you through a four-phase plan to help you make important changes to restore vibrant health.

Everyone needs to understand what causes chronically high insulin levels and type 2 diabetes, and we need to learn how to eat to keep blood sugar levels in the safe range. The Reclaim Diet puts that information into your hands, and it is proving to be a more powerful tool than medication. The answer is not the latest fad diet, weight loss pill, exogenous ketones, or eating less and exercising more.

What is the answer?

The answer lies in first breaking food addictions, shunning highly processed foods, reducing the intake of insulin-spiking carbohydrates and flooding our bodies with nutrient-rich unprocessed real food. The Reclaim Diet puts valuable, life-changing, practical information into your hands.

The Reclaim Diet is not a short-term fad diet but a four-phase plan to help you redeem your life and rescue you from a destiny of chronic disease, over-medication and food obsession. Briefly, here are the four phases.

Phase 1: Elimination. A 30-day real food plan called the elimination diet to quickly identify foods that are causing unwanted reactions in your body. In phase 1, you will learn how to flood your body with real-food nutrients and break common addictions to processed food.

Phase 2: Reintroduction. A systematic plan to guide you through testing foods that were removed during Phase 1 to determine if any foods are problematic for you. During Phase 2, continue to follow the elimination diet while you add in one new food every three days.

This phase typically takes a few weeks. At the end you will know how well you tolerate common allergenic foods like wheat and other grains, dairy, corn, and soy.

Phase 3: Individualization. While continuing to eat a real-food diet, using the information you discovered in Phase 2, you will be able to customize the plan and relax the strict rules from the elimination diet. This is not a return to your former ways. You will have been healing your body, reducing chronically high insulin levels, and enjoying a state of reduced inflammation. Through Phase 1 and Phase 2, you will discover how food has been contributing to your health problems, and more importantly, how certain foods create a feeling of well-being and satiety as you experience new levels of vibrant health.

Phase 4: Lifestyle. We are all different and there is no one-size-fits-all diet. You will keep the concept of eating real food as your foundation. The Reclaim Diet is not a fad diet that you start and stop. This is the healthy human diet—based on eating real food, including the right amount of protein, healthy fats and nutrient-rich, colorful vegetables and fruit, with seeds and nuts. You will decide, based on the information I provide around food quality and on your personal health goals and belief system, what foods you will allow back in, how often, and how much. This will be the time when you will be in a better place to implement concepts like intermittent fasting. And, ultimately, you will be creating a lifestyle that is sustainable and enjoyable.

Stay curious and reclaim your health

Stay curious and be open to the idea that you can recalibrate your life. You can take steps beginning today to recover health and wellness. Be willing and open to new possibilities that may have been hidden from you until now.

Nutrition science is evolving, with take-away messages that are conflicting and seemingly get more and more complicated. For example, humans happily consumed eggs for several thousand years until we became smart and figured out some of the nutrients in an egg included cholesterol and fat. Well meaning scientists and doctors told us to take eggs off the menu because they wrongly believed that the cholesterol in the egg would somehow create heart disease. Twenty years ago, a very large study involving 118,000 people concluded that eggs can be eaten every day and eggs do not increase the risk of coronary heart disease and stroke (9).

In April, 2019, apparently without digging into the details, Dr. Oz fell for the "clickbait" headlines, "Study Puts Eggs and Dietary Cholesterol Back on the Radar (10)." Oz reported to his followers, "Clearly, more than one egg yolk a week could scramble your health. Here's a smart alternative: Stick with cholesterol-free egg whites and veggies for a tasty omelet (11)."

If Dr. Oz had looked at how the study was conducted, he would have seen that it was not an actual controlled study, but data taken from several large groups of people who had filled out food frequency questionnaires. Data may have been collected every four years from these groups, at best. People in the groups had to recall how many eggs they ate and how often. If people reported they ate eggs, the researchers tried to find a correlation directly to heart disease and all causes of death, 17 years later. We don't know what else the study participants ate—it could have been a diet of eggs, Honey Buns and Twinkies. Did they smoke, drink too much, exercise too little or have too much stress? The study claimed to find a weak correlation between egg consumption and poor health outcomes.

Correlation is not causation. That is like correlating the fact that everytime there is a home that catches fire, firemen are mysteriously at the scene. Firemen are not causing fires, and eggs are not causing heart disease.

This example is to highlight the importance of not being gullible to "clickbait" headlines and junk science. Data can be manipulated and exprapotolated and misused. Seeing people's lives restored through dietary and lifestyle change is powerful, but science says these are anecdotes and they don't count. Thousands of anecdotes matter. Eric Westman, MD, a physician, researcher and director of Duke Lifestyle Medicine Clinic said, "I believe clinical observation is evidence. In fact that's the history of clinical epidemiology starting with the evidence of what you see in your clinic." (12) Dr. Westman has been using a low-carb approach in his clinic for over 20 years, and I have been helping people for almost that long with a real food, low-carb approach.

You know how they say, "When the student is ready, the teacher will appear." Who knows that you haven't stumbled upon this book at the exact moment that you need it, or maybe it was a gift from a caring friend. Maybe this is the answer that you have been looking for.

Here is Jim's story. He needed answers and serendipitously ended up attending my class, Achieving Wellness and Weight Loss. Jim's friends wanted to help him learn how to change the way he was eating when he was diagnosed with type 2 diabetes.

Jim lost 45 pounds and dropped his blood sugar 300 points

Jim Okrzesik was diagnosed with type 2 diabetes at age 53, after experiencing dramatic drops in energy, disorientation, increased thirst and increased urination.

His doctor prescribed a statin drug (to lower cholesterol) and sent him to see a dietitian. Unable to get an appointment for six weeks, Jim's friends brought him to a class I was teaching. I explained to the class the importance of eating unprocessed whole food.

I suggested a plan based on eating three meals a day. Each meal was to include quality animal protein, healthy fat and plenty of non-starchy vegetables. Jim began to eat grass-fed meat, wild-caught fish, pasture-raised chickens and eggs when possible. He included healthy fats like butter, extra-virgin olive oil and coconut oil. Jim increased his intake of colorful vegetables.

In two months, Jim's blood sugar dropped from over 400mg/dl to an average of 90 - 115 mg/dl, without medication. He lost 45 pounds and his pants size dropped from a 38- to 32-inch waist.

Health tip to try today: Add one tablespoon of raw apple cider vinegar to six ounces of water and consume before meals. Raw apple cider vinegar improves the action of insulin in the body and can reduce post-meal blood sugar levels in people with type 2 diabetes (13, 14). Rinse your mouth after consuming vinegar.

CHAPTER 3

EVERYTHING I THOUGHT I KNEW
ABOUT FOOD WAS WRONG

How would you answer this question if I asked, "Do you eat a healthy diet?"

Ninety-percent of Americans believe their diet is good, very good or excellent, according to a survey by Consumer Reports®. Most people believe that they are making healthy choices, but they are comparing their diet to the wrong standard.

We have come to believe that the government has been giving us good dietary recommendations over the last 50 to 100 years. If these recommendations were right, we would not be witnessing the current devastating degradation of the nation's health.

- 1 in 10 U.S. adults have diabetes, the CDC reports. If current trends continue, 1 in 3 U.S. adults could have diabetes by 2050.
- 2 in 3 adults are overweight or obese (National Health and Nutrition Examination Survey).
- 1 in 4 people die from heart disease.
- 1 in 6 people suffer from chronic constipation.

Most Americans believe that all they need to do is eat less and exercise more to lose weight. Most people believe that they are eating a healthy diet if they are eating exactly what their doctors and the government tell them to eat.

Let's take a moment to think about these questions.

- You want to eat a healthy diet, don't you?
- Where can you learn HOW to eat a healthy diet?
- Who can you trust?

Can we trust the government to give nutrition advice?

Every five years, the U.S. Department of Health and Human Services (HHS) and the U.S. Department of Agriculture (USDA) jointly publish the *Dietary Guidelines for Americans*. Their goal is to make recommendations to promote health, prevent disease and help people reach and maintain a healthy weight.

Good luck trying to read the 95 page document which includes six chapters, charts, tables, definitions, Appendix 1-15, and tired advice that does not work.

To improve health and lose weight, the *Dietary Guidelines for Americans* provide an endless list of vague or confusing rules:

- cut calories and exercise more
- reduce sodium to less than 2,300 mg (unless you are African American, have high blood pressure, diabetes or kidney disease)

- eat no more than 10% of calories from saturated fats
- consume no more than 300 mg per day of cholesterol
- limit your trans fats
- reduce your solid fats
- reduce added sugars
- limit consumption of refined grains, but half of all grains should be whole grains
- increase your intake of low-fat dairy
- increase your intake of fortified soy beverages
- emphasize vegetables, fruits, whole grains, fat-free or low-fat milk products, seafood, lean meats and poultry, eggs, beans and peas, and nuts and seeds

In the end, the USDA tried to simplify a healthy diet by giving us the silly MyPlate program. It is completely out of balance because it was influenced by the agriculture industry. MyPlate recommends that over 75% of the food is carbohydrates, less than 25% is protein and 0% is fat, with an unknown portion of dairy is recommended.

Does the American Diabetes Association (ADA) understand nutrition?

The ADA says it is ok for diabetics to eat whole-grain pasta, cereal, bread, beans and fruit (including dried and canned) with other foods—just "find the right balance."

Unfortunately, when we eat one cup of pasta, two cups of cereal and two pieces of bread in one day, those foods are highly processed and turn into 35 teaspoons of sugar in your blood.

Here's how to easily calculate how much sugar your food turns into:

- Add up the total carbohydrates (grams) in the food you are consuming.
- Divide the total carbohydrate grams by four.
- That number equals the number of teaspoons of sugar being dumped into your bloodstream.
- Here's an example. Thomas' cinnamon raisin bagel has 56 grams of carbohydrate. 56 divided by four equals 14. Eating this bagel spikes your blood sugar with the equivalent of 14 teaspoons of sugar.

I do want to commend the American Diabetes Association for appointing Tracey Brown in 2018 as their new chief executive. Tracey is the first-ever CEO of the ADA to be living with diabetes. She has said publicly that she was diagnosed with type 2 diabetes 15 years ago and is now eating a low-carbohydrate diet. Tracey has been able to come off insulin and three other medications by being mindful about sugar and carbohydrates. I encourage you to watch Tracey's video interview with journalist Stephanie Gaines-Bryant, of the Sisters4Fitness podcast, dated January 28, 2020.

I was impressed with Tracey Brown's commitment to communicating a truthful and inspiring message. I hope that her experience and knowledge will bring needed change to the current ADA dietary recommendations.

Can we trust the nutrition advice from the Academy of Nutrition and Dietetics (formerly known as the American Dietetic Association)?

This group recommends the USDA's MyPlate program mentioned earlier. This Academy believes that we should consume grain foods like oats, brown rice, or whole-grain pastas, breads and cereals.

This group, according to their 2015 annual report, has taken money from corporate sponsors like Coca-Cola Company, Splenda®, General Mills, Kellogg Company, PepsiCo, Campbell Soup Company, Premier Protein®, and Conagra. Of course, the Academy of Nutrition and Dietetics recommends products from their sponsors, and they will not speak the truth about sponsors' health-damaging processed foods.

Do we need the government or pharmaceutical-funded interest groups dictating to us what constitutes a healthy diet?

How were you taught to eat?

When I was in school we were taught to eat according to the USDA "Basic Four" food groups:

1. Vegetables and fruit

2. Milk, including cheese and ice cream

3. Meat

4. Cereal and breads, including pasta, cereal and rice

My grade school did not offer hot lunch, so I walked a few blocks to eat lunch at home. More often than not, my lunch was a bologna sandwich on white bread and Campbell's bean soup. If I brought my lunch to school, I could buy a carton of milk and a cup of ice cream (checking off two from the dairy group).

Processed and fast food dominated the sixties and seventies. Pop Tarts or cereal with milk for breakfast—actually, I didn't like to pour milk on my Sugar Frosted Flakes, because I was worried that the sugar would wash off.

We ate a lot of canned food like Chef Boyardee or Campbell's Chunky Soup with little "sirloin burgers" for our meat. We ate a lot of scrambled eggs and toast for a quick dinner. Sometimes we had beef or pork, with a side of canned vegetables or iceberg lettuce salad with Thousand Island Dressing. My grandma made us casseroles using noodles, sour cream and canned soup. We all thought we were eating a healthy diet because we hit the Basic Four food groups, sort of.

The Basic Four was released in 1956, and the focus was on getting enough of certain foods. It was not designed for building health and preventing chronic disease, and Americans' health was spiraling downward by following these recommendations.

Our government purposefully buried solid nutrition advice to help industry.

In the 1980s, the government hired a team of top nutritionists to revamp the 1956 recommendations. This group, led by Luise Light, dug into scientific research for months and produced a solid plan which included these daily recommendations:

- 5 - 9 servings of fresh vegetables and fruit (the base of the pyramid)
- 5 - 7 ounces of protein foods like meat, eggs, nuts and beans
- 4 tablespoons of added fat from cold-pressed fats like olive oil and flaxseed oil
- Strictly limit refined carbohydrates and sugar (use sparingly: bread, rolls, crackers, candy and junk food)
- Keep grains to a maximum of 2 - 3 servings per day, always in whole form

This plan developed by the team of nutritionists never saw the light of day.

Luise Light, the nutritionist who led the team that developed the first version of the food pyramid described above, said, "When our version of the Food Guide came back to us revised, we were shocked to find that it was vastly different from the one we had developed. As I later discovered, the wholesale changes made to the guide by the Office of the Secretary of Agriculture were calculated to win the acceptance of the food industry."

The revised guidelines were not at all in line with what the nutritionists recommended:

- Processed foods were emphasized over fresh and whole foods.
- The servings of wheat and other grains were dramatically increased to make the wheat growers happy.
- Refined grains—including crackers, sweets and other low-nutrient processed grain foods—were moved from the top of the pyramid to the base.
- The recommendation for 5-9 servings of fresh fruits and vegetables a day was slashed to just 2-3 servings. Later it was changed to 5 - 7 servings.
- Instead of a maximum intake of 3-4 daily servings of whole-grain breads and cereals, the government decided to up this to a whopping 6-11 servings to appease the processed wheat and corn industries.

Luise Light said, "I vehemently protested that the changes, if followed, could lead to an epidemic of obesity and diabetes—and couldn't be justified on either health or nutritional grounds. Over my objections, the Food Guide Pyramid was finalized. Yet it appears my warning has come to pass."

The food industry is shaping the government's food advice.

The government revamps its food guidelines about every five years and continues to give harmful and deceptive advice that protects interest groups in the food industry. These recommendations have little to do with providing Americans with valid health and nutrition advice, and everything to do with making a profit.

Following the government's dietary guidelines is making us a sick and fat nation.

As a result of twisted politics and profit-driven motives, in 1992 the USDA handed us the misguided MyPyramid. They decided to be very specific with the number of servings we were told to eat and had food icons in the diagram.

The MyPyramid recommendations were not based on nutritional science:

- 6 - 11 servings of bread, cereal, rice, pasta, crackers
- 2 - 4 servings of fruit
- 3 - 5 servings of vegetables
- 2 - 3 servings of milk, yogurt, cheese
- 2 - 3 servings of meat, poultry, fish, eggs, dry beans, and nuts
- Use sparingly: Fats, oils, sweets

"It is not based on any nutritional science. It is not based on any clinical or medical observations. It has been created by politicians who are protecting the interests of the wealthy," said Dr. Natasha Campbell-McBride, a medical doctor with two postgraduate degrees: Master of Medical Sciences in Neurology and Master of Medical Sciences in Human Nutrition.

Neurologist calls the food pyramid a perverse recommendation for human health.

David Perlmutter, MD and Board-Certified Neurologist, said, "We created this higher carbohydrate, lower fat/calorie idea which was called, here in America, the Food Pyramid, which was the most perverse recommendation for human health that has ever been conceived."

We all have been following dietary guidelines that keep us sick.

You and I have been following the government's dietary guidelines for most of our lives. My kids grew up with MyPyramid and their schools followed this model.

I had to stop letting my daughters buy lunch at school because the choices were so unhealthy, even though they met all the requirements of the USDA guidelines. The school menu items listed Corn Dogs, Pizza, Sloppy Joes, and "Walking Taco" (which I think was a bag of Fritos with meat tossed in). The sides were overcooked green beans, corn, peas, and tater tots.

I followed the Food Pyramid at home. Even though I thought I was making a better quality meal for the family, I was not. I fed my family boxed macaroni and cheese, spaghetti with Prego, pot pies, tacos made with seasoning packets, boxed cereal, bread, pudding, Jell-O, chips, juice, chicken nuggets, cookies, and pizza—just like everyone else I knew.

The kids were little when we moved from the Midwest to California, and I tried to help the family eat better, but I really wasn't sure what that meant. Sun Chips® instead of Doritos®? Whole-grain bread instead of white? Cheerios™ instead of Fruity PEBBLES™? Whole-wheat pasta instead of regular? I was confused.

The turning point for me came when my health started deteriorating. The earliest symptoms I had were panic attacks and optic migraines. Later, I developed chronic hives, and I just wanted someone to tell me what to eat to make the horrific itching stop and get the unsightly welts to disappear forever.

My poor, life-long decisions around food led to my health problems, and I came to learn that food would get me out.

Following the dietary recommendations handed down from the government will surely make us all chronically sick. Eating primarily unprocessed foods, like quality meats and fish with healthy fats, vegetables and fruit, restores health.

I also learned this the hard way: If you go back to eating the Standard American Diet (even if your health was previously restored from eating unprocessed, real food), you will go back to the same old health problems.

I am teaching you the way out, and I promise it will not be a confusing list of hard-to-follow rules.

The truth is most people do not realize that they are eating foods that feed cancer, cause weight gain, and promote inflammation, the condition that is the common thread of all the major chronic diseases.

Wouldn't you love to stop chasing diets and counting calories, and start loving your food and how it makes you feel? This is going to be fun, and I just know that if you follow these recommendations, you will reclaim your health.

Are you hesitant to try this eating plan?

Sometimes people are skeptical about trying the Reclaim Diet plan and making a lifestyle change over to unprocessed food. Ann was very hesitant to change the way she ate, but she was desperate and willing to give it a try to resolve chronic headaches, fibromyalgia, pain, fatigue, brain fog and blue moods.

"Erin helped me get my life back when I was feeling so bad and didn't know why. Changing to 'real' food changed my life!"

Ann shared, "I had several chronic conditions including daily headaches for four months that I had seen a chiropractor, acupuncturist, physical therapist and medical doctor for. I was taking pain medication daily. I had been diagnosed with eczema several years ago, and was recently experiencing hives. I was also battling fibromyalgia. I suffered from muscle aches, joint pain, fatigue, "tired" eyes, lack of concentration and brain fog. I'd been on antidepressants for many years.

I had already made an appointment to see a brain surgeon for my headaches, but Erin encouraged me to try her plan first. I agreed to follow the plan and I eliminated all food allergens while eating unprocessed foods like animal protein, vegetables, fruit, healthy fat and nuts. I felt pretty lousy on day two and day three, but to my surprise, by day five I felt like a new person.

I had more energy, no more "tired" eyes, joint pain, muscle aches or brain fog. I couldn't believe how my concentration improved. I could read something and actually remember it. I was amazed at how my mood had improved. I felt so happy. I have since been able to decrease my antidepressants. My skin issues and headaches took about one month to go away, and I very rarely now experience them.

Since I've changed my eating habits, I feel like a new person when I exercise. My muscles actually work like they are supposed to—no joint or muscle pain, and no fatigue afterward. My muscle strength and range of motion has improved a lot.

I could never have imagined what a difference eating the right foods could make in my life. My quality of life has truly improved since I started eating "real" food and staying away from the food that my body is sensitive to. I'm so thankful to Erin for suggesting this diet to me and helping me so much along the way with encouragement and recipes." — Ann Beatty

It has been 10 years, and Ann is still feeling fantastic as she continues to follow the real food plan.

Health tip to try today: Assess what percent of your diet is processed food from a package or can by writing down everything that you consume for a few days. Today, we have access to many processed foods that are promoted as healthy options. They may be marketed as sugar-free, fat-free, low-carb, paleo, grain-free, or keto. These foods include bars, candy, breakfast cereal, desserts, chips and crackers. Move away from expensive, processed food and focus on including more unprocessed food—fresh produce, meat, fish, chicken, eggs and nuts.

CHAPTER 4

GET YOUR LIFE BACK ON TRACK, THE BEST IS YET TO COME

- ✓ How do you change life-long habits that have resulted in a sick body?
- ✓ How do you ditch the beloved, addicting foods?
- ✓ When will you start seeing results?

Like me, you want to get better. I remember thinking, "Just tell me what to do, and I'll do it!" Once I found a functional medicine doctor to help me, I jumped in with both feet. While I know you are anxious to get to the plan and start experiencing results, you do not need to feel overwhelmed with a long list of things to change. This book will give you a step-by-step plan that you can use to work at a pace that is comfortable for you. I encourage you to add one positive step after another until you find success and a lifestyle that is helping you achieve your health goals.

In addition to giving you a step-by-step plan, I want to help you gain an understanding of why so many people are suffering and struggling with health these days. I will weave in the foundational information along the way, giving you things to do to start moving the needle. There is no 30 Day Reset or Miracle Diet of the Month. You are looking for more. You are looking for a sustainable plan that will become your new lifestyle. You are ready to get your life back.

It starts with a choice.

You made the choice to find and purchase this book, so you are already on the journey and ready to experience new levels of health and wellness. What would your ideal healthy self look like? Here are a few areas where people see a positive shift as they implement the plan:

- *Energy.* Energy to wake up easily, and not crash mid-morning, mid-afternoon, or after dinner.
- *Sleep.* Enjoying deep, restful sleep without medication and alcohol.
- *Weight.* Feeling comfortable with the process of achieving your optimal weight.
- *Hormones.* Good hormonal balance is more than optimizing sex hormones and includes managing hormones associated with stress and blood sugar.
- *Mood.* Having even moods without wild, uncontrollable swings.
- *Brain.* Your brain is focused, calm and clear, allowing you to enjoy life and accomplish your goals.

"I have a whole new lease on life!"

Stephanie noticed a change in her moods. She felt "off" and "spaced out" for over eight months. She made an appointment with a psychiatrist who didn't spend any time talking with her but simply said, "What drugs do you want? I'll fill your prescription."

"When I met with Erin back in January, I felt horrible. I felt totally hormonally out of whack. I cried easily, couldn't focus, was tired, moody, heavy and bloated. I wasn't sleeping well, and I felt like it was totally out of my control. Now it's like I have a whole new lease on life! I've lost weight (25 pounds) but more importantly, I feel balanced and healthy and in control of my health and wellness. I thought menopause doomed me and was making all the decisions. I'm still working on everything, but WOW what a difference this eating plan and essential oils have made! God put Erin in my path, and I am grateful." — Stephanie A.

When it comes to your health, are you frustrated with where you are right now?

Do you find yourself chasing after grocery store magazine diets that promise a quick fix? Do you revert back to the low calorie, high exercise plan to lose weight?

That plan does not work, and it will never work for long term, sustained weight loss.

I am going to help you cut through all the conflicting messages out there to find a new level of health and wellness that you desire. You can have a renewed hope for the future, no matter where you are beginning this journey and no matter how many times you have failed. I am confident that the essential plan that I have developed will give you exactly what you need to fix your health naturally.

Are you ready to move away from the SICKcare model that has led to a nation of people who are mostly fat, sick and tired?

Do you believe that chronic disease can be prevented and sometimes even reversed? I believe that making diet and lifestyle changes can eliminate the risk factors of many chronic diseases, and I am not alone.

"In reality, the major causes of chronic diseases are known, and if these risk factors were eliminated, at least 80% of all heart disease, stroke and type 2 diabetes would be prevented; over 40% of cancer would be prevented." — The World Health Organization

Health tip to try today: What would your ideal healthy self look like? If you had a magic wand and could change anything about your health, what would be three to five items on your list? Would you like to reduce or eliminate certain medications? Would you like to sleep like a baby and lose weight effortlessly? Are you concerned that you see your energy levels declining? The human body is resilient, and can heal in ways that often surprise people. We have to do our part to eat nourishing food and live a healthy lifestyle, and this may mean letting go of conventional dogma and being open to trying something new. Without putting any limitations on yourself, what would you like to change about your health?

CHAPTER 5

LEAVE THE PAST BEHIND, IT'S A NEW DAY!

If you feel frustrated that, no matter what you do, it seems like your weight keeps increasing and your health and energy keep decreasing, you are not alone.

Are you tired of trying new plans and feeling paralyzed by all the possibilities? Are you confused by conflicting health advice?

My hope is for this book to help you make new discoveries and give you hope and encouragement that will keep you moving forward on your health journey.

As long as we are alive, health is a journey, not a destination.

You can always be moving forward if you are willing to seek new paradigms and new truths, while letting go of old ways that are not working for you.

If it seems like there is a wall or barrier that is preventing you from getting your life back, don't rule this out: the wall may be guiding you off your current path. The barrier on your path may be telling you that it is time to take a turn and gain a new perspective on how to lose weight, boost energy, sleep better, and reclaim your health.

A common wall that everyone faces is the Standard American Diet.

The Standard American Diet (SAD) is creating a downward spiral of weight gain and chronic illness. As a society, we have been drifting way off the course that served us well for thousands of years. Over the past 100 years, our food supply and what we eat has changed dramatically. We switched from eating fresh whole foods high in nutritional value to consuming processed foods that are convenient and easy. Mass-produced food manipulated for a long shelf life, with cheap ingredients and eye appeal, actually contains health-damaging ingredients and has little nutritional value.

You can dramatically change all aspects of your health by ditching processed foods, grains, sugar, soy and commercially produced milk products. You can do this, and I will walk you through. Maybe you cannot do everything all at once but you can take baby steps in the right direction. Don't hesitate to start small, because motion leads to momentum.

In this book, you will learn how to stop yo-yo dieting and how to stop making unhealthy choices. I will show you how to start healing your body and metabolic rate so that you can look and feel amazing.

You want to follow a plan that gets results, but one that is healing and sustainable as well. You will learn that fixing health naturally is not hard and eating real, unprocessed, food is enjoyable. While some people are ready to jump in with both feet and start experiencing results, you are free to learn and add one positive step after another until you find success and a lifestyle that serves you well. So, are you ready to reclaim your life and start on your health journey? Let's get started!

"I'm down 30 pounds and rarely have cravings"

Heidi joined my online community, Whole Healthy Journey. After following the plan, Heidi reported to the group on her progress. "So it's an anniversary of sorts—one year ago I started on this real food plan. I couldn't be more grateful for the ways it has helped me in ways I didn't even know I needed.

I'm sure I'm not doing everything right, but I try and I have stuck with it. Though I know it's not all about the weight, I'm down 30 pounds, rarely have cravings, not groggy in the afternoons, no deep hunger feelings, skin and hair are fantastic.

I would really like to lose just a little more but I've been the same for quite awhile now so I think those last few pounds just love me too much to ever leave me. I've yo-yo dieted my whole life, so I will not starve myself to lose the weight. This plan is for real. Thanks, Erin!" — Heidi C.

Health tip to try today: Join our online Facebook community, Whole Healthy Journey, today. Enjoy reading the posts and take a look at the files for the group to grab some free recipes and helpful information.

PART II

THIS IS WHY YOU ARE SICK

Part 2 Introduction

One of your most important healing tools is the correct nutritional approach. I have seen it time and time again for nearly two decades; people can fix a lot of their health problems with good, whole-food nutrition.

Before you go counting calories, it's more important to first eliminate any foods causing a negative effect on your body. These include foods that are causing an immune response. That means your immune system may be on defense alert to certain foods preventing you from enjoying the quality of life you desire. I will help you figure out which foods are triggering an unwanted immune response.

Do you get seven or eight hours of restorative sleep? Lack of sleep, too much stress and exposure to harmful chemicals in our everyday products are all important factors that can keep you from experiencing health and vitality—regardless of diet.

In Part 2, we will explore some of these important topics and help you learn how to make some simple but powerful changes that will make a significant difference in your health.

CHAPTER 6

CALORIES COUNT ... OR DO THEY?

Do you count calories? If so, you are likely wasting time you could be spending on gaining optimal health.

Sick of yo-yo diets? The media and food brands have been lying to you. They want you to fill your body with low-calorie, nutrient-defunct foods that will do nothing to help you optimize your weight for the long-term. You may find that every time you diet it is harder and harder to lose weight and impossible to maintain.

Many women I counsel confess to being life-long dieters. During their diet, they will feel hunger and cravings constantly. While they may lose weight initially, they damage their metabolism and are unable to get off the diet without the weight coming back quickly.

If you're struggling to understand how to reach an optimal weight and feel healthy and vibrant, it's not your fault. There are many factors at play and it can be difficult to understand how they work together. That's where I come in :). I will teach you how to determine which foods are causing problems and why. I will also guide you on how to know which foods are your friends and which foods are your worst enemies.

Weight Watchers, Atkins, Mediterranean—there's so many diet plans out there, how can they all be right? The truth is, they're not.

In fact, what most people believe to be true about weight loss is the very thing that keeps them from achieving wellness and hitting their weight loss goals.

I am referring to the common belief in the CICO model. You know—calories in, calories out. Some people use this for weight loss but it is, at best, an inadequate tool if your goal is to fix your health naturally and optimize your weight in a sustainable way.

All calories are *not* the same, so it doesn't make sense to focus on just calories.

Are all calories equally fattening? No. A calorie of Doritos® is not the same as a calorie of spinach.

A cup of spinach is seven calories, which is filling, thanks to the fiber. Plus spinach is rich in vitamins, minerals and a wide variety of nutrients.

Seven calories of Doritos® is not filling. It is less than two whole chips. Chips are full of genetically modified (GMO) corn and sugar, inflammatory vegetable oils, artificial dyes, MSG and preservatives that deplete health.

Calories count, but this is not the most important parameter for improving health and achieving optimal weight. Many people like the simple concept of counting calories because it is easy to measure and track. But one problem with using the energy equation is that you need to understand what "calories out" means. It is not simply the number of calories reported by your treadmill after a workout.

We expend calories walking, breathing, digesting food, and all the things our body does to keep us functioning. When we eat whole foods, more energy is required and more calories are expended than when we consume the same calories of processed food.

Eating a piece of salmon or the same isocaloric (same number of calories) amount of a baked potato will have different effects in the body. The starchy potato is a fast-acting carbohydrate. It causes a rise in insulin that results in negative metabolic effects. The salmon will not have that effect. Eating salmon is more satiating, so you will feel satisfied for a longer period of time.

In 2009, a Scandinavian study had people eat similarly with the exception of snacks. One group snacked on fast-acting carbohydrates (candy) while another group snacked on an isocaloric amount of peanuts (mostly fat and protein). The study lasted two weeks and the snacks were added to their regular diet.

The group snacking on fast-acting carbohydrates **experienced more weight gain and waist circumference increased significantly**, even though the calories stayed the same. LDL cholesterol and ApoB numbers were higher, indicating less favorable metabolic health.

On the other hand, the metabolic rate increased for those subjects snacking on peanuts, but **those participants did not gain weight or increase the size of their waist**. What this shows is that the body does not treat all calories equally. It is not as simple as calories in equals calories out (15).

Other studies have compared low-carbohydrate diets to low-fat diets to show that reducing carbohydrates is more effective for weight loss and fat loss than a low-fat diet (16, 17).

There are many popular diets, like the Mediterranean diet and the low-fat diet, that leave you feeling hungry because they focus on foods that are less filling.

I find that people want to eat the right foods but get confused by conflicting messages. Is a plant-based diet best? Is red meat and saturated fat harmful?

I, like many of you, grew up believing that the USDA Food Pyramid was a healthy model. I ate 6-11 servings of grains and bought as many fat-free products as I could find. Most of the food I purchased was processed and convenient. I ate bread, cereal, pasta, tacos, chips, pizza, sandwiches, fruit, and very few vegetables.

While I was not overweight, my health was slipping away. My doctors were offering more pills, but no real solutions. Fortunately, my sister, Chris, encouraged me to make an appointment with osteopathic physician Dr. Joseph Mercola. He was the physician that guided me through my health challenges using whole foods, including healthy fats and animal foods as well as vegetables, fruit, seeds and nuts.

Seeing my body respond and heal as I incorporated healthy foods was life changing for me. I chose to pursue a master's degree in holistic nutrition education so that I could help people who are struggling with health and weight issues. One person, Kris, found me by reading success stories on my website. Here's her story.

Kris tried to do "clean eating" but would fall off the wagon and feel frustrated.

Stubborn health challenges had plagued Kris for a long time.

She described herself as "very overweight" and had a long list of health concerns:

- Fibromyalgia
- Rosacea
- Stress
- Heart Palpitations (her doctor did an EKG and said she was fine)

Kris just wanted to feel better and start turning the weight around.

By following my plan, she began eating flavorful, delicious foods that were more nutritious and more filling. Kris loved eating this way and began to see results.

As the months went along, Kris reported that she was feeling so much better. All of her symptoms were decreasing rapidly and her body was healing. She was dropping weight, and no longer felt inflamed. In just five months she lost 50 pounds without even thinking about calories.

By following my plan, Kris found out that she was reacting to certain foods. She began to eat nutritious foods that reduced inflammation in her body and in her skin. Discovering which foods she was sensitive to gave Kris key information that she needed to begin turning her chronic health problems around. In the next chapter I will help you understand how food sensitivities may be ruining your health.

Health tip to try today: A few years ago, I challenged a group of 40 people to take my water challenge for 30 days. At the end of the challenge, participants completed a survey. The results were astounding:

- Digestion improved
- Joint aches and pains were reduced
- Brain function improved (stable moods, mental clarity, headaches resolved)
- Skin appearance improved (more hydrated, softer, reduced blemishes)
- Energy increased
- Sleep improved
- Weight loss experienced without dietary changes
- Hunger and cravings reduced

I challenge you to give it a try! For 30 days, drink 24 ounces of purified water upon rising. During the day, consume about two quarts of water or half your body weight in ounces of water. For example, if you weigh 180 pounds, drink 90 ounces of water. Do not drink anything during meals, and be sure to add high quality mineral salt. Read the details on my blog at:

GetBetterWellness.com/waterchallenge/

Chapter 7

Undiscovered food sensitivities may be ruining your health

Food Allergies and Food Sensitivities

Did you know that the foods you eat could be causing your body to react with an unwanted immune system response?

You may be aware of people with food allergies to nuts or shellfish, for example. When exposed to these foods, the reaction may be immediate, severe and potentially life-threatening. The cause of the severe allergic reaction is from the immune system overreacting by producing IgE (immunoglobulin E) antibodies. If you have IgE food allergies, you probably discovered this by now and take precautions.

Food sensitivities, on the other hand, are different. You may not be aware that you have them. Instead of triggering an immediate reaction, these sensitivities typically involve a delayed immune response (triggering the IgG immune reaction in your body). It may take from one to three days for symptoms to present.

It is very common for people to have a sensitivity to common foods like dairy, corn or gluten, the protein found in wheat, barley, rye and other grains. Whether or not you have digestive symptoms, food sensitivity symptoms are numerous and can affect all parts of the body. Scientific papers list dozens of symptoms connected to gluten sensitivity, including neurological symptoms, digestive symptoms, recurrent ear infections, daily headaches, sleep problems, behavioral issues, hallucinations, abdominal pain and weight changes.

Apathetic 14-year-old girl with anxiety, crying spells, hallucinations and insomnia gets off two anti-psychotic drugs after changing her diet.

This story is about a 14-year-old girl who had been perfectly fine up until age 12 when she started having daily headaches and difficulty concentrating. She started to have difficulty sleeping, and her behavior at home and school worsened. She had crying spells and was unmotivated and apathetic. Doctors prescribed the anti-anxiety medication bromazepam.

Instead of seeing improvement, the girl started to have hallucinations, lose weight and experience bloating and constipation. Doctors admitted her to a psych ward and performed a battery of lab tests, but most were normal. A year later when her symptoms worsened, she was prescribed another anti-psychotic drug.

Finally, two months later a nutritionist was consulted and a gluten-free diet was recommended. Within a week the girl experienced a dramatic improvement in both intestinal and psychiatric symptoms. Her doctors tested her for a wheat allergy (IgE) and performed several tests, including a skin prick test to wheat. The girl tested negative for all common allergy tests.

Her parents chose to start the girl on a strict gluten-free diet and the girl experienced complete regression of all symptoms within a week. The doctors helped her stop the medications they had prescribed and the mother recalled that she was returned a "normal girl." Nine months after starting the gluten-free diet, she remains symptom-free (18).

It is sad that this girl suffered for years and was misdiagnosed and prescribed dangerous medication that even gave her suicidal thoughts. The crime is that food was not considered until long into the process. This is a great example of SICKcare in this nation, and we can change that thinking today.

What are your symptoms telling you?

While this constellation of symptoms in one person may seem like an unusual reaction to gluten, I ask you to consider that your symptoms may be related to an intolerance to gluten or other foods like dairy, soy, corn and additives in processed food.

Celiac disease (CD) is an autoimmune reaction to gluten but only 1 to 3% of the population have CD. In autoimmune conditions, the immune system attacks the body's tissues. The symptoms are terrible if it is not treated. People experience an inflammatory immune response that may manifest as chronic diarrhea, constipation, weight loss, bloating, abdominal pain, indigestion and nutritional deficiencies. The symptoms can affect any organ or tissue in your body.

People may not absorb iron and be diagnosed with anemia. Without adequate absorption of nutrients, CD can lead to bone loss, joint pain, dementia, seizure, infertility, numbness in the hands and feet and even schizophrenia. Removing gluten turns the disease process off, according to Dr. Alessio Fasano, a well-known researcher in the fields of celiac disease and gluten intolerance (19).

Just because you don't have celiac, doesn't mean you are not reacting to gluten.

As I mentioned, there is another common problem people experience that is a reaction to gluten called gluten sensitivity. This is not an allergy or an autoimmune condition. It is an immune reaction that can cause inflammation in the intestines or elsewhere in the body.

Clues that you are gluten sensitive or have CD:

- Digestive symptoms (bloating, diarrhea, constipation)
- Abdominal pain
- Brain and neurological symptoms (brain fog, lack of focus)
- Headache or migraines
- Joint and muscle pain
- Arm or leg numbness
- Anxiety and depression
- Hormonal imbalance
- Liver problems
- Circulatory system problems
- Acne

- Skin rashes (hives, eczema, psoriasis, idiopathic dermatitis, alopecia areata)
- Dermatitis herpetiformis (bumpy, itchy, burning rash with blisters)
- Nutritional deficiencies
- Anemia
- Fatigue
- Unexplained weight gain or loss

You may experience any of those symptoms above if you have a sensitivity to gluten, dairy, soy, corn, other gluten-free grains, legumes, eggs, citrus, yeast or nightshades (tomato, potato, eggplant, peppers).

How to discover which foods cause unwanted reactions for you

The best way to discover which foods are causing a reaction in you is to complete a 30-day plan, commonly called the elimination diet. I think that the "elimination diet" needs a new marketing team, don't you? We might be drawn to the plan if it had a more appealing name, but it is a very powerful, life-changing tool that we all can use, because it is free. This is an eating plan that includes unprocessed, anti-inflammatory, healing real food. The key to experiencing powerful results lies in the handful of foods that are eliminated 100% for 30 days. I will share the details with you in Part 4.

Health tip to try today: Keep a food journal.

For now, an easy step is to start paying attention to how certain foods make you feel. Keeping a simple food journal can be eye-opening. Write down everything that you eat and drink for a few days. Note how you feel after eating. Are you sleepy or more alert? Does it feel like food is sitting in your stomach? Do you feel satisfied after a meal, or do you crave something else? What are you craving and when do you feel the cravings?

A food journal is most beneficial during the elimination diet and the phase that follows, the reintroduction period. Right now, if you are still eating wheat, dairy and corn you may not know why a meal containing cheese pizza and corn on the cob made you feel terrible. During the elimination diet, you will know if it was wheat, dairy, corn or all three, because of the systematic way we check each food.

CHAPTER 8

INFLAMMATION: THE ROOT OF ALL DISEASE

10 common causes and the top 10 anti-inflammatory foods to include today

Do you have any of the following conditions or symptoms?

- Joint pain
- Muscle pain
- Asthma
- Psoriasis
- Sinus problems
- Migraines
- Crohn's disease
- Heart disease

There's a common thread to these chronic conditions – inflammation.

Pain and inflammation are signals that you might be doing something wrong. The body produces pain and inflammation temporarily so that you will go find the cause and fix it. The SICKcare model offers quick fix drugs in order to medicate away the symptoms and reduce the pain without dealing with the root cause.

Inflammation plays a major role in these and many other conditions. If you have arthritis or psoriasis, the inflammation is fairly obvious. Your joints are painful or your skin is inflamed. But, you also may be dealing with hidden inflammation which can be just as dangerous since it is degrading your health every day without you even knowing it.

Hidden inflammation may be connected to heart disease, dementia, and digestive problems.

Inflammation is your immune system reacting to injury or infection as a way to help you heal. If you get a thorn in your finger and your finger turns red and puffs up, that is inflammation that we can see. When you are fighting a sore throat you may notice your throat is red and swollen. This type of inflammation goes away; it is beneficial and it is short-term.

Some inflammation is chronic. There may be irritation and inflammation inside the body. We don't see it but it can cause major problems.

Here are some results of inflammation in the body:

- Inflammation in the blood vessels could lead to heart disease.
- Inflammation in the brain can be short-lasting or it may be long-lasting, continuing to cause damage that leads to dementia and Alzheimer's disease.
- Brain inflammation can also result in brain fog or headaches and loss of energy.

- Whole-body inflammation is a long-term, inflammatory response throughout your whole body. You may feel pain everywhere, or it may be simmering in the background. An abnormal lab test for C-reactive protein may be your first indication of systemic inflammation.

We want the body to produce an inflammatory response for acute problems like microbes and injury. It is the long-term, chronic inflammation that is keeping you feeling unwell. Thankfully, this is often within your control.

Getting your life back means increasing your awareness of what causes inflammation so that you can address and fix the root cause.

The top 10 triggers of controllable inflammation

1. **Inflammatory foods.** Eating foods that cause a sensitivity, allergic reaction or inflammatory response.

2. **Poor Diet.** Eating a poor diet high in processed foods, sugar, conventional meat, pasteurized dairy, refined grains and common cooking oils.

3. **Dehydration** from too little clean water and too much caffeine, alcohol and soda.

4. **Environmental toxins.** Exposure to harmful chemicals in food and water from pesticides, herbicides and heavy metals.

5. **Harmful chemicals.** Allowing harmful chemicals to get into our bodies through products we use around our homes (cleaning

chemicals, lawn care, insect sprays, air fresheners) and in our personal care (toothpaste, shampoo, soap, lotion, perfume).

6. **Obesity and overweight.** Inflammation is a consequence of being overweight and obese which may lead to a number of chronic diseases (20).

7. **Alcohol.** Drinking too much alcohol weakens the immune system making it vulnerable to inflammatory conditions of many body systems (21).

8. **Stress** can be emotional, psychological or physical. Your body responds by raising your stress hormone, cortisol, and creating inflammation.

9. **Medication.** Over-the-counter and prescription pharmaceutical drugs cause an inflammatory response in the body. Most of these medicines and drugs are synthetic and primarily derived from petrochemicals (22).

10. **Poor sleep.** Lack of adequate, restful sleep triggers inflammation (23).

The Reclaim Diet Plan will start to cool the fires of inflammation caused by most of the top 10 triggers listed above.

Your food choices play a large part in whether or not you are experiencing inflammation. When your internal fires of inflammation are burning, you are more likely to gain weight and have poor health.

As you become more aware of how certain foods make you feel and understand the connection between inflammation and processed food, begin to focus on adding anti-inflammatory foods into your diet.

Add in these top 10 anti-inflammatory foods.

While the Reclaim Diet helps you move away from some of the top ten triggers of inflammation, it is time to add in powerful foods to combat inflammation and flood your body with healing nutrients.

Choosing to eat the right anti-inflammatory foods helps reduce the risk of illness and disease.

1. **Leafy greens** like chard, collard greens, dandelion greens, kale, beet greens, mustard greens, parsley and spinach are rich in phytochemical with anti-inflammatory properties and anti-cancer properties. Vary the greens that you eat and eat some raw and cooked greens. Including a healthy fat will increase the absorption of nutrients.

    - For a delicious side dish, sauté greens in butter, add onion and garlic, and season with salt and pepper.
    - Make kale chips. Tear a large bundle of kale into pieces, coat with 2 Tbsp avocado oil or coconut oil, season with salt. Experiment by adding 1 tsp chili powder or 1 Tbsp nutritional yeast. Bake at 250 degrees for 15-20 minutes, watching so they do not burn.

2.   **Ginger** has potent compounds called gingerols that have been shown to be helpful for swelling and joint pain.

- Steep half-inch slices of fresh ginger in a cup of hot water to make ginger tea.
- Regularly add fresh, grated ginger to salads, stir-fry, marinades and other foods to enjoy the anti-inflammatory and germ-fighting benefits.

3.   **Allium vegetables: Onions and garlic** are the most popular in this family, but others to include are leeks, scallions, chives and shallots. These foods have sulfur-containing compounds that provide health benefits and an anti-inflammatory and immune-boosting effect. Interesting to note that red onions have twice as many antioxidants as other onion varieties and are powerful foods for inflammation.

- Choose garlic bulbs and onions for the most flavor and health benefits. Onion and garlic powder and jars of crushed garlic and pre-cut onions are convenient, but they miss the mark on nutrition compared to preparing your own at home.
- If you dread cutting onions because it irritates your eyes, try chilling the onion for an hour before cutting and use a sharp knife.

4.   **Turmeric root** has curcumin and has significant anti-inflammatory benefits. It is as potent as many anti-inflammatory drugs.

- Try making the anti-inflammatory beverage called Golden Milk. Blend 1/2 tsp organic turmeric, 1/2 tsp cinnamon, 1/4 tsp ginger, 1 cup warm (canned) coconut milk and a dash of pepper. Add a little raw honey or liquid stevia if desired.
- Sprinkle turmeric on eggs, vegetables, and add to homemade soups and sauces.

5. **Beets** have compounds that help fight inflammation, protect cells, and improve cardiovascular function. Beets are unique because they are a great source for betalains, plant compounds that have antioxidant, anti-inflammatory and detoxification properties.

- Avoid long cooking times to keep the betalains from being damaged.
- Cut medium beets into quarters. No need to remove the skin before steaming. Steam for 15 minutes. Rub the skin off with a paper towel.
- Grate raw beets for salads or use to garnish soups.

6. **Berries and cherries** contain antioxidants that have anti-inflammatory effects. Eating berries, pomegranates, wolfberries, acai, elderberries, and cranberries helps fight inflammation and reduces the risk of cancer and heart disease.

- Buy organic, frozen mixed berries and add to a smoothie.
- For a healthy dessert, try 1/2 cup frozen berries, slightly thawed, topped with 1/3 cup canned coconut milk. Sprinkle with nuts, ground flax seeds or shredded coconut.

7.   **Pineapple** has a powerful enzyme, bromelain, known to decrease inflammation and help with bronchitis, sore throats, sinusitis, arthritis and sports injury. It also helps prevent swelling after trauma or surgery. The highest concentration of bromelain is in the core of the pineapple. Eating pineapple between meals will maximize bromelain's effects. I save the pineapple core in freezer bags and add pieces to smoothies.

8.   **Fatty fish** (wild-caught salmon, sardines, cod, tuna). These foods are rich in the omega-3 fatty acids, DHA and EPA, which are known to support the immune system and help with inflammation.

- Shopping tip: Choose wild-caught fish instead of farm-raised fish. Wild-caught fish come from seas, rivers and natural bodies of water. Farm-raised fish come from tanks and enclosures within bodies of water. The fish are often vaccinated and may have more toxins than wild-caught fish. Farmed fish are often fed an unnatural diet of corn and soy so they are less nutritious.

- Quick-broil fish: Coat fish with avocado oil, season with salt and pepper. Preheat an oven-safe skillet (stainless steel or enameled cast iron work well) under the broiler for 10 minutes. Add fish to the hot pan, return to broiler and cook for about 5-7 minutes depending on thickness. This method cooks the fish rapidly on both sides.

- Season fish with anti-inflammatory herbs and spices like ginger and turmeric (great for joint pain). Try different anti-inflammatory herbs and spices like basil, rosemary, thyme, oregano or adobo.

9. **Sprouted pumpkin seeds** are a powerhouse of antioxidants that support health and reduce inflammation. Sprouted pumpkin seeds have been soaked (for easier digestion) and dehydrated to activate their full potential. They contain 7 grams of protein per ounce and are a good source of vitamins and minerals like zinc and magnesium.

- I like the brand Go Raw for organic sprouted pumpkin seeds with only a little Celtic sea salt added.
- Add to salads or enjoy as part of a homemade trail mix.
- Add sprouted seeds to smoothies.
- If you have a food processor or VitaMix, blend 3 cups sprouted pumpkin seeds into a wonderful, smooth seed butter. Warning, your processor may not be up to the task! If your machine is heating up, stop, take a break and come back after it cools down.

10. **Bone broth** is easy to make at home (see my recipe at GetBetterWellness.com). Homemade bone broth is a great way to ease inflammation and joint pain. The nutrients are beneficial for skin, hair and nail growth, and known to help heal the digestive tract and calm the mind.

- Drink a cup or two of bone broth every day.

- Use bone broth to make soups and stews.

- Ease pain and inflammation with this delicious recipe, Golden Turmeric Broth. Simmer together in a small pot: 2 cups bone broth, 1/2 cup canned coconut milk, 1/2 tsp turmeric, 1/2 tsp ground ginger, 1-2 cloves crushed garlic, 1/8 tsp pepper and unrefined salt. If you prefer, remove the garlic with a spoon before drinking.

Keep this list handy and include a variety of anti-inflammatory foods to your Real Food Plan every day.

Cecelia followed my Real Food Plan and experienced life changing results.

"Following Erin's recommendations, I lost 30 pounds, [and] rid myself of panic attacks, hair loss, massive pain in my body, numbness in my face, swelling in my neck and chronic inflammation! I was told that I had MS, but by just changing the way I ate, all the symptoms went away completely! I now have more energy than I have had in years and feel fantastic everyday.

"This isn't a quick fix diet pill, but Erin teaches you what our toxic American diet does to our bodies and how to transform your health from the inside out. She teaches you the skills you need to transform your health and to get your body to crave good food so that you can get off the junk food train! You will not regret incorporating this information into your life.

It will save you lots of money down the road in doctor bills and medications! Blessings, Cecelia Bruce."

Health tip to try today: Incorporate anti-inflammatory foods every day.

Review the list of the top 10 anti-inflammatory foods above. Choose to add at least one food every day. Experiment with some of the recipes and ideas in the list.

CHAPTER 9

THREE ENERGY ROBBERS THAT STEAL MORE THAN YOUR ENERGY

On a scale of 1 to 10, how would you rate your energy?

- Do you wake up ready for the day (10) or do you have difficulty waking up and dragging yourself out of bed (1)?

- Is your energy pretty good? Does it feel even all day long (10) or you need caffeine and sugar during the day to get moving and stay alert (1)?

- Do you fall asleep easily and sleep deeply for seven or eight hours without the help of alcohol or medication (10) or do you feel wired at the end of the day and need a cocktail or a glass of wine, or two, to wind down before bed (1)?

- Do you have enough energy in the evening to do light chores, engage with family and friends, read or watch a movie (10) or do you fall asleep on the couch after dinner (1)?

If your energy scores are not 35 to 40, your body is not functioning the way it was designed to. Once you start eating according to the real food plan, your body will start to come back into balance, and you will LOVE how you will feel.

Take a hard look at some of these energy robbers. If your total score was between 4 and 20, you are not alone. Only one in seven Americans report waking up feeling refreshed every day, according to a poll conducted by YouGov.com.

While there are many reasons that you may feel exhausted, you may be eating foods and drinking beverages that cause an energy drop, resulting in unwanted fat storage.

What are the top three energy robbers?

Here are three energy robbers that may be stealing your energy and causing you to have mood swings, brain fog, haywire hormones, faster aging skin and unwanted fat storage.

1. The Blood Sugar Roller Coaster

Are you on the blood sugar roller coaster?

- Do you have to eat every 2 hours?
- Are you constantly snacking and grazing?
- Do you get shaky, angry, and feel like you are starving if you don't eat for a few hours?
- Do you have an energy slump after lunch requiring coffee, soda or a sugar treat to get you through the afternoon?

Sweeteners, grains, processed foods, refined flour, excess fruit and starchy vegetables are carbohydrate foods that convert into too much sugar in your bloodstream. Consuming these foods may be putting you on the blood sugar roller coaster.

The blood sugar roller coaster is stressful for your body.

The spikes in blood sugar are followed by crashes that cause your body to release the stress hormone cortisol. Over time, having high cortisol levels at the wrong time can deplete your happy brain chemicals, interrupt sleep patterns, kill brain cells and cause you to store more belly fat.

We want to eat carbs that come from non-starchy vegetables mostly with some whole fruit, seeds and nuts. Processed grains like bread, bagels, cereal, pasta, crackers and chips are turning into lots and lots of sugar and putting you on the blood sugar roller coaster.

How many teaspoons of sugar do you consume daily? You may be surprised by how much.

If you are curious how much sugar your food turns into, take the total number of carbohydrate (grams) and divide it by 4. This will give you an approximation of how many teaspoons of sugar will be in your bloodstream after each food you consume and digest.

Here are some examples of common foods and how much sugar enters your bloodstream after you consume them.:

- Bagel - 56 grams carbs - 14 tsp sugar
- Starbucks Eight Grain Roll - 68 grams carbs - 17 tsp sugar
- Old Fashioned Oatmeal, 1.5 cups cooked - 50 grams - 12.5 tsp sugar
- Fiber One Cereal Honey Clusters, 1 cup - 44 grams carbs - 11 tsp sugar

- Spaghetti, 2 cups cooked - 86 grams carbs - 21.5 tsp sugar
- McDonald's Medium Fries - 48 grams carbs - 12 tsp sugar

According to Michael R. Eades, MD, a normal fasting blood sugar represents less than 1 teaspoon of sugar dissolved in the blood. So when you eat a Starbucks Eight Grain Roll in the morning you are getting 68 grams of carbohydrates which converts to about 17 tsp of sugar. Your blood sugar will spike and then drop within a few hours. You will feel the drop in energy and that leads to a craving for more carbs and sugar.

Eating a low-carb breakfast changes this pattern and gives you a stable source of energy.

For example, a two-egg omelet cooked in butter and prepared with one cup of vegetables, served with 1/2 cup of blueberries on the side is only 18 grams of carbs. Plugging 18 grams into our simple equation we see that this healthy breakfast turns into just 4.5 tsp sugar.

You will feel full, satisfied and well-nourished when you eat quality **protein**, healthy **fat** and plenty of **vegetables**. I will refer to this magical meal combo of protein, fat and vegetables as PFV. Always build meals around PFV first, then add 1/2 cup of berries or other fruit, if you like.

You are not spiking your blood sugar, you are not crashing after this breakfast and you are not storing belly fat like you would with a high carb meal of bread and cereal. Instead of beginning the day with no food or eating starchy, processed food, try eating a breakfast with protein, vegetables and berries. You will love how your energy and hunger levels remain stable all day long.

2. The Morning Beverage Addiction

Coffee and certain morning beverages can be a pleasure, a ritual, a habit and possibly an energy robber. Drinking too much coffee, let's say more than 20 ounces a day, may not be beneficial.

Caffeine is a stimulant that increases your heart rate, blood pressure and anxiety levels. If you are using caffeine to prop yourself up during the day, then this is going to be an energy robber for you and may be the reason why you cannot get a good night's sleep.

Here's the good news about coffee:

Coffee can be healthy and is a great source of antioxidants. Coffee can boost your metabolism and help with weight loss and fat burning. Studies show that coffee drinkers have less calcium deposits in their arteries (24), and, for people who tolerate it, coffee has many benefits for the brain (25).

Not all coffee is healthy for you.

Mass-produced coffee has adverse health effects from pesticides and the presence of mold toxins. Coffee is sprayed with more chemicals than any other product consumed by humans, next to tobacco. If you want health benefits from drinking coffee it will be easier if you avoid Folgers, Maxwell House, Starbucks, grocery store brands, Dunkin' Donuts and McDonalds.

Opt for organic, shade grown coffee.

Shade grown coffee is most often organically grown without chemicals. Mass-produced coffee is sun grown, which is a process that depends on pesticides and chemical fertilizers and is destroying the environment.

When looking for organic, shade grown coffee, two brands that I trust are Purity Coffee and Myorga Organics.

Drink good coffee, not "froofie" coffee from the coffee shop.

If you are going to drink coffee or a caffeine beverage, keep in mind that the coffee shop options are not typically offering organic coffee. Often coffee shops are brewing inferior, sun grown coffee and they are adding sweeteners, artificial flavors, gums, preservatives, trans fats and low-quality dairy.

Going back to the first energy robber, the blood sugar roller coaster, these sugary coffee drinks are a nightmare for depleting health and packing on the pounds.

For example, a Frappuccino Blended Coffee is full of unwanted ingredients and has 72 g of carbohydrates, dumping 18 teaspoons of sugar into your bloodstream.

Your coffee habit may be sabotaging your efforts to improve your health and lose weight.

Purchase organic coffee beans and brew coffee at home.

Skip the highly refined sweeteners, and especially skip the flavored creamers. I like using a handheld immersion blender to whip in organic butter, canned coconut milk, or for an extra brain boost with weight loss benefits, MCT oil. Add 1-3 tsp of MCT Oil (I love the brand, Kiss My Keto, C8 Brain Fuel) and blend. If you are new to MCT, begin with 1 tsp and slowly work up to 3 tsp to let your body get used to this new fat.

3. Alcohol - The Calm Before the Storm

If you are a teetotaler, meaning you totally abstain from drinking alcohol-containing liquids, then this section does not apply to you. If you enjoy a glass of wine or other alcoholic beverage now and then or even every night, then consider that this energy robber may be robbing more than your energy in ways that might surprise you.

Why you wake up between 2:00 and 3:00 a.m. after drinking alcohol

When consuming alcohol in any amount, people typically fall asleep easily for the first half of the night. Somewhere around 2 or 3 in the morning your body becomes more active as it needs to process the alcohol. Your heart rate increases, which leads to an increase in night sweats and urination. Alcohol disrupts your normal sleep cycle, and you will feel more tired the next day.

Can alcohol cause nocturnal leg cramps?

Alcohol causes dehydration, depletes key vitamins and minerals and leads to an increase in lactic acid. You are more likely to experience nocturnal leg cramps in the muscles of your feet, calves and thigh.

The cramps can last for a few seconds or a few excruciating minutes and, just as you fall asleep again, you may be hit with another painful cramp. These cramps can be very severe. Your body will handle it eventually, but the cramps may last for minutes or sometimes several hours.

Fat burning is paused.

Alcohol disrupts fat burning. Your body knows that alcohol is a toxin and it will abandon other functions to work on the alcohol. Many people want to believe that the only problem with drinking alcohol is the carbs. While carbs are a valid concern, drinking alcohol can also affect your ability to maintain good health, sleep well, experience healthy energy levels and avoid nasty leg cramps.

Don't worry, I am not asking you to be a teetotaler.

Here are some ideas to help you reel it in if you feel like you are consuming too much alcohol. If you are tired of not sleeping well, getting leg cramps and feeling frustrated with the fat growing around your midsection, try these tips below to help manage your alcohol intake:

- **Be honest with yourself** and keep an accurate record for a few weeks of exactly how much alcohol you are consuming. Record total ounces, not glasses. At the end of each week try to associate the amount of alcohol with a financial value. You might be surprised to see how much you are drinking and how much money is being spent on alcohol over the month.

In terms of alcohol content, 5 oz of wine equals 1.5 oz of spirits. Beer typically has gluten, the inflammatory protein in wheat and other grains. Beer can sabotage an otherwise healthy journey.

- **Alcohol-free nights**. Because we know that alcohol interferes with sleep cycles, it is important to keep the majority of your nights alcohol-free. Drinking wine every night might have health benefits if you are drinking one glass of red wine with dinner. The reality is that one glass often becomes two glasses, and before you know it, you are consuming a whole bottle every night.

- **Accelerated aging**. Too much alcohol is going to age you faster, disrupt your plans for a flat belly, increase your risk of breast cancer (26), deplete your body's glutathione (master antioxidant that detoxifies harmful substances), and harm your liver. Spend most of your nights abstaining, rather than drinking.

- **Water before bed**. When drinking wine, it is best to drink it with dinner and then switch to drinking water before bed. How much wine is too much? The benefits won't likely become harmful if you drink only one or two glasses of red wine, up to three or four nights a week, and abstain from excessive drinking on any one night.

- **Don't get caught in the justification trap**. Stop making little deals with yourself. Do you find yourself justifying drinking too much ("I was good all week, so I can have four drinks on Saturday") or promising to do better on Monday morning? Alcohol is trapping you.

- **Go cold turkey**. Completely eliminating alcohol from your diet can give you your power back. How long does it take? That depends on you. Maybe you just need to stop and never drink again. Maybe you can stop for 30 days and then come back as suggested, with a glass of red wine at dinner, then switching to water and having more alcohol-free nights during the week than nights with alcohol. When people follow this eating plan and get off the blood sugar roller coaster, they experience many surprising health benefits. One man, Steve, shared what happened after he and his wife, Cindy, learned how important it is to stop consuming foods that quickly convert into sugar.

"I lost 30 pounds and I have a more consistent feeling of higher energy throughout the day with little or no afternoon slump."

"Erin's class was just what my wife Cindy and I needed. A few habits and health issues were causing me some concern and the information I learned confirmed what I had been suspecting for some time. The class gave us both the jolt we needed to make changes in our eating. Over the years, I had accumulated four or five prescriptions. With some research, I started to suspect that one drug was leading to another. I was taking a statin, a few medications for high blood pressure, something for heartburn/reflux, and most recently Metformin for type 2 diabetes. Then doctors discovered polyps in my colon and I was having IBS symptoms! What next? I discovered that the statin can lead to diabetes and the Metformin can mess with your colon!

"I experienced good results from a few years of following Erin's recommendations of low carb eating. With some reading, my wife's encouragement, and Erin's advice, I quit all my prescription drugs. I just quit all of it! My doctor does not know all of this, yet. My next appointment is soon, but from my point of view, it's going great! My blood glucose is almost normal—I test it often at home to monitor how my body is responding to certain food. I don't know about my cholesterol, but I've learned that the whole statin obsession is more about making money and managing numbers than building health.

"I don't have reflux anymore—I started intermittent fasting, and I don't eat as much. I have lost over 30 pounds. That in turn improves all the numbers. My blood pressure still seems to run a bit high, but more exercise and sticking with real food should continue to bring that down. I have a more consistent feeling of higher energy throughout the day with little or no afternoon slump. I am in my late 60s and, all in all, I'm feeling better than ever. Hopefully, my doctor will agree, and give more credit to building health rather than managing illness!" — Steve Nelson

Health tip to try today: Fix breakfast!

Instead of skipping breakfast or running out the door with a granola bar and coffee, plan time into your routine to prepare a low-carb breakfast, like I described above in the section on the blood sugar roller coaster. If cooking eggs in the morning seems daunting, then make an egg bake ahead of time. For a variety of recipes, google the phrase "paleo egg bake" or "paleo breakfast casserole" to find recipes that can be made in a 9x13 dish ahead of time. Then just reheat a piece to start your day with ease. I suggested the search term "paleo" because that is the easiest way to find recipes that are free from common allergens, like wheat and milk products. If your go-to egg casserole includes bread and cheese, I encourage you to try something new!

Chapter 10

Four Reasons That You Need About Eight Hours of Sleep

Are you sleep deprived and sick?

If your life is busy and full of responsibilities, you might be like 40% of Americans who are running on less and less sleep. If so, you are "sleep deprived" and part of what the Centers for Disease Control and Prevention labels as a public health epidemic.

Pay attention "night owls" — this is what you may be unknowingly signing up for:

- Depression and mood disorders
- Crankiness and emotional outbursts
- More hunger, overeating and weight gain
- Decreased immune function
- Slow digestion with more constipation
- Increased risk of type 2 diabetes
- Increased risk of cardiovascular disease
- Development, promotion, and progression of cancers from light at night, disrupting melatonin production (27)
- Less brain detoxification, increasing the risk of dementia
- Shortened life expectancy
- Increased accidents and death from drowsy driving

Without enough sleep, we all become tall two-year-olds.

— JoJo Jensen, *Dirt Farmer Wisdom*, 2002

No matter how hard we try, we cannot trick the body. We cannot "get used to" sleeping less without suffering health consequences. A recent study found that one night of poor sleep could create insulin resistance, the situation that opens the door for weight gain and diabetes (28).

Yes, even you, superwoman, need eight hours of sleep.

While children of school age need 10 or more hours of sleep, adults need at least seven and probably eight hours of sleep each night (29).

Here are a few reasons to help motivate you to get more sleep:

1.   **You will burn more fat and calories and desire to eat fewer carbs and less food** (30).

- The fat-burning growth hormones spike during deep sleep. You will notice a difference in your ability to lose fat and increase muscle growth when you prioritize sleep.
- Cut yourself short on sleep and you will gain weight and store fat more easily.
- Proper sleep keeps levels of the stress hormone, cortisol, in check. Less cortisol means less belly fat.
- Lack of sleep can have unwanted effects on your sex hormones.

2. **Magic melatonin increases.**

Melatonin is the sleep hormone that regulates your body's sleep-wake cycles. It works in darkness, not while you stare at the television or an electronic device.

Adequate melatonin has many benefits in the body (31):

- Inhibits oxidation and inflammation
- Helps fight against liver injury
- Protects the brain
- Cardioprotective: melatonin protects against various heart diseases
- Reduces sensitivity to pain
- Reduces anxiety
- Antineophobic - this is just a big word that means melatonin helps you deal with new situations, places or things
- Eases depression
- Reduces blood pressure
- Fights tumors
- Benefits eye and blood vessel health

3. **Your brain will have a fantastic tune up.**

Your brain wants you to sleep and will reward you when you do (32).

You will be able to:

- Think clearly
- Retain and remember information

- Make decisions
- Solve problems
- Improve school and work performance
- Feel more creative and have new ideas

"Sleep is important for mental function: alertness, memory consolidation, mood regulation and physical health," says Phyllis C. Zee, MD, PhD, professor of neurology and director of the Sleep Disorders Center at the Northwestern University Feinberg School of Medicine in Chicago.

4. **You will be healthier overall and your skin will thank you.**

When you sleep, your body repairs and rebuilds and protects itself from illness:

- Cells are renewed
- Everyday damage from free radicals is reversed
- Your skin loses the sallow, dehydrated look
- You lose the puffy eyes and dark circles

These ten tips will have you sleeping better in no time.

1. **Eat well.** A real food diet with quality animal protein, healthy fat, vegetables, fruit, seeds and nuts will help balance hormones and will help you sleep better. Avoid processed foods which are loaded with refined carbohydrates and hidden MSG that can leave you feeling wired.

2. **Have a healthy bedtime snack.** The right snack will help maintain your blood sugar levels while you sleep, especially during Phase 1. Sugary sweets, chips and simple carbs lead to a drop in blood sugar which causes you to wake up. Try half an apple with a tablespoon of almond butter or sunflower butter; or guacamole with vegetables.

3. **Commit to getting on a schedule.** Go to bed and get up at the same time each day to create a good rhythm for your body. Aim for seven or eight hours of sleep. Turn down the thermostat at bedtime.

4. **Start your day with sunshine** and take Vitamin D3 with K2. Sunlight in the morning helps balance sleep-wake cycles. Try to go outside in the morning for 15 minutes, without sunglasses and without a hat. Go for a quick walk or sit on the patio. Keep this habit up, even on cloudy days, and you will find that your sleep will begin to improve.

5. **Limit or avoid electronic usage** one to two hours before bed. Electronics disrupt sleep patterns and melatonin production needed for sleep. You might also want to install an application that tints your screen to neutralize the blue light. Resources include f.lux, Redshift, or Night Shift (built into iOS).

6. **Dim the lights in the evening and consider wearing blue light-blocking glasses.** Swannies glasses from Swannick Sleep are a good option to block blue light.

7.   **Enjoy a bath with Epsom salts and essential oils.** Epsom salts provide the calming mineral magnesium that your skin absorbs. Add essential oils like lavender to enhance the relaxing benefits. A drop or two of essential oils applied to the bottoms of the feet before bed will be quickly absorbed and help promote deep, restful sleep. I love the combination of Tangerine, Orange, Ylang ylang, Patchouli, and Blue tansy essential oil. It is appropriately named, Peace & Calming®, and is beneficial to quiet children down at night, too, so you can get some rest.

8.   **Take magnesium glycinate capsules at bedtime.** 300 to 600 mg before bed will help you relax and fall asleep.

9.   **CBD tincture** can be taken under the tongue before bed to assist with sleep. In the resources section, I have more educational information on CBD and choosing quality products.

10. **Use melatonin** to break bad patterns or to avoid feeling jet lagged. Taking four or five milligrams of melatonin at bedtime encourages a restful night's sleep.

Brian lost 20 pounds and after following my real food plan for four months, he no longer needed a CPAP machine.

Brian's wife often complained about his snoring. Brian knew he was waking up several times during the night and never felt rested or refreshed in the morning. He was drinking coffee and Diet Coke to stay awake at work.

When he started falling asleep Brian's doctor had a sleep study done and was diagnosed with sleep apnea and given a CPAP machine and mask to wear while he slept. When Brian's wife started following my nutrition advice, he went along and liked eating real, unprocessed food. "My body enjoyed the food," he said. Brian began eating a healthy breakfast with protein and vegetables, he cut out fast food and bread and stopped drinking soda. Brian lost 20 pounds, and after following my real food plan for four months, he no longer needed the CPAP machine.

Health tip to try today: get a good night's rest.

If you are not sleeping for seven or eight hours each night, take a look at the ten tips above and try a few of the suggestions.

Part III

Time to Embrace a New Way and Experience Change that Heals

CHAPTER 11

WHEN YOU ARE SICK AND TIRED OF FEELING THE WAY YOU DO, CHOOSE A NEW APPROACH

Maybe I should have suspected that a life built on cereal and English muffins, Big Macs and French fries, spaghetti and Reese's Peanut Butter Cups was going to catch up to me one day. I was shocked when seemingly overnight my health started changing. Dealing with anxiety and panic attacks, chronic hives, and a diagnosis of Hashimoto's thyroiditis made me wonder, "Why is this happening to me?"

I tried medication but felt really frustrated that doctors were not treating me as a whole person. Instead, I was referred to several specialists. The endocrinologist gave me Synthroid, but no advice on diet. The dermatologist gave me several prescriptions for hives, and also thought I needed an antidepressant, but he never talked with me about my diet. My gynecologist gave me a prescription for Xanax, gleeful that he knew how to stop my panic attacks. Again, not one doctor asked me what I was eating.

Thankfully, out of this growing frustration, I was beginning to listen to my sister's advice. Maybe I needed to find a new doctor who could advise me on food and supplements. I had little faith that this natural approach would work, but I was willing to try. In fact, I decided that I was going to be the model patient, because I was sick and tired of doctors and prescriptions that were not helping me.

Physicians lack nutrition training in medical school.

A study published in 2010 highlighted the fact that while patients routinely seek nutrition and diet advice from physicians, little priority is given to nutrition education for physicians in medical school. Practical advice on healthy diets is barely addressed and most medical schools give less than 25 hours of training over the five or six years of education (33).

This miracle prevents 1 in 5 deaths every year, without side effects.

It is a crime that our physicians are not given nutrition education and are ill-equipped to share powerful, life-saving information with patients. A study published in *The Lancet* showed that if people were to eat a nutrient-dense diet,   this step alone could prevent 1 in 5 deaths every year (34).

The best thing we can do to heal ourselves is to forget the biased USDA information that created the Dietary Guidelines. Instead, we should return to a traditional diet and nourish ourselves with delicious, nutritious and satisfying foods. In 2007, 11 million deaths were attributed to poor dietary choices. Are you on track to be a statistic like I was?

Today, a gift is before you. It is the opportunity to change the path that you are on. You may be at a fork in the road right now trying to decide if you will stop eating the Standard American Diet and return to eating a traditional, whole food diet. I encourage you to choose to be 100% all in so that you can enjoy 100% of the benefits. Are you ready to dive in and get more into the details of this way of eating? First, let's highlight a few health benefits this way of eating brings.

Ten benefits you can enjoy when you eat real food

1. **Optimized weight.** Not everyone needs to lose weight. You may be at your ideal weight or even below, but eating this way will optimize your body composition and weight.

2. **Increased energy.** The cells that make up every organ and tissue in your body have powerhouses inside them called mitochondria. Every cell (except red blood cells) can have anywhere from 1 to 2,000 mitochondria, that each have multiple "batteries" inside (35). Mitochondria turn nutrients and oxygen into energy. When you want to feel more energetic all day long, feed your powerhouses by eating a nutrient-rich diet. Enjoy a rainbow of fresh vegetables and fruit, quality animal protein, and healthy fats. Eating processed foods, grains and sugar is like feeding sludge to mitochondria, leaving you tired and lethargic.

3. **Improved sleep.** Sleep is a gift and it is during this time that our body heals and repairs itself. The first step to improving sleep is to address nutrition. Eating foods that boost the sleep hormone melatonin is a natural way to help regulate your circadian rhythm. Regularly eat the following foods shown to contain melatonin: meat (beef, lamb, pork), poultry, eggs, fish, nuts, seeds, mushrooms,

strawberries, tart cherries, cranberries, garlic, onion, ginger, tomato and the Chinese wolfberry (36).

4. **Better hormonal balance.** One of the ways we can improve hormonal balance is with nutritious, unprocessed food. Eat high-quality protein and unrefined fats to give your body what it needs to support hormone production. Regularly include grass-fed meats and butter, wild-caught salmon, coconut oil, avocado oil, pastured eggs and olive oil.

5. **Elevated moods.** Diet and nutrition are critical in balancing moods. We need to eat adequate, quality protein to give our body the building blocks needed to make neurotransmitters, our happy brain chemicals. We need to make sure our digestion is working well, since 95% of the body's serotonin is housed in the gut (37).

6. **Improvement in chronic health conditions.** When we eat a traditional diet, foods that our ancestors ate before we had modern farming and food processing, our bodies will gain the building blocks that support good health. Replacing processed foods that sabotage health with nutrient-dense foods will allow the body to heal. People usually experience dramatic improvements in blood sugar, blood pressure, digestion, pain, skin rashes, brain fog and inflammation.

7. **Reduced belly fat.** Following the Standard American Diet has resulted in more belly fat for Americans. No matter how many crunches you do, eating too many sugars and processed foods will create unwanted body fat. The foods that promote the accumulation

of belly fat include sugar, high fructose corn syrup, grain-based foods (like bread, pasta, cereal, crackers and chips) and inflammatory processed foods. To increase fat-burning, focus on eating vegetables, protein and healthy fats.

8. **Reduced cravings and hunger.** Many people eating the Standard American Diet are familiar with cravings and extreme feeling of hunger accompanied by compulsive thoughts about food when a meal has been missed. Contrast this to people eating a grain-free, whole-food diet who report a reduction in food cravings and an increase in satiety (38).

9. **Increased enjoyment of food.** When people incorporate quality protein, fat and plant foods into their meals and pull out the processed foods like bread, crackers, chips and other packaged foods, they will experience an awakening of taste buds. Once your body adjusts to eating whole, unprocessed food, you will appreciate and enjoy eating this way and notice a greater satisfaction with food.

10. **Break sugar addictions.** Most people know that they should eat more vegetables and whole foods, but they feel powerless when it comes to sugar. Over the years, I have helped many people break their addiction to sugar in as little as seven days. The secret is to add in a bounty of vegetables, animal protein and healthy fats at least three times a day and make a serious commitment to avoid all sugar and grains for seven days. You can do that! Just imagine that I was going to pay you $1,000,000 just for eating grain-free, sugar-free and processed-food-free for one week. I know you would be successful

and when you can get through seven days without those foods, the grip that sugar seems to have on you will loosen. Each day you will realize how fabulous you are feeling, and how amazingly quiet your cravings have become.

The best way to optimize weight and health is to eat real food.

I have my clients and everyone in my coaching groups begin the same way, PFVx3 (PFV times 3).

PFVx3 simply means eat **P**rotein, **F**at and **V**egetables at each of three meals daily. That is easy to remember, right? A PFV breakfast might be a veggie omelet cooked in healthy fat with a side of organic sausage. For lunch you might opt for a big salad with lots of colorful vegetables. Include 3 or 4 ounces of beef, chicken or fish. Add a good dressing made with olive oil and toss in some fresh avocado for additional healthy fat. When preparing dinner, it is easy to plan to have some sort of meat, fish or chicken with two types of vegetables. Roasting vegetables in avocado oil or coconut oil is a delicious way to incorporate more vegetables into your day.

Choosing whole, unprocessed foods is the key to being a healthy human. When it comes to sourcing food, buy the highest quality that you can afford. It is a myth that eating whole foods needs to break the budget. When money is not being spent on soft drinks, juice, chips, crackers, bread, treats, cereal and pasta, you will have the funds needed to put towards healthy, unprocessed foods. I recorded two podcasts that will give many practical tips to help you eat well on a budget. Find them on iTunes or Blog Talk Radio. My show is called,

Fixing Healthy Naturally with Erin Chamerlik.

- How to do Real Food in the Real World
- Paleo on a Budget for Families

Have you been frustrated with feeling sick and tired and not getting any answers?

Maybe it is time to try a new approach. That's what Kathy did, and it turned her 10-year health battle around. Here is the story that Kathy shared with me recently.

"I was gaining weight uncontrollably. I had sores all over my arms, sinus infections, wheezing from uncontrolled asthma, kidney stones, arthritic pain, brain fog, and severe pain and edema in my feet and ankles. My hormones felt completely out of balance. I could not sleep, yet I felt fatigued all day long and battled anxiety and depression.

"My friend Lonna introduced me to Erin because I was sick—really sick—and tired and frustrated. Doctors told me there was nothing wrong with me, but my symptoms were mounting.

"The education that Erin provided me was life changing. I learned that certain foods I was eating were causing many of my symptoms and allergies (even though doctors tested me and said I did not have any food allergies).

"Erin introduced me to REAL food, meaning unprocessed, whole foods with one ingredient. Initially I removed gluten from my diet.

While this relieved many symptoms it was not until I removed all grains and dairy and stopped eating processed foods that I felt significant improvement in all areas of my health. I no longer need multiple medications for asthma. No more allergy shots, pills, nasal sprays, or asthma inhalers. I no longer need Ibuprofen to deal with swelling and pain.

"By testing my saliva hormones, we learned that my adrenal glands were suffering and contributing to my fatigue and hormonal imbalance. Erin put together a protocol for me that included lifestyle changes, supplements and bioidentical progesterone.

"For ten years, I felt like I lost my ability to enjoy life fully, but now all that has changed. I was sick and tired of being sick and tired and Erin helped me find the way out. Following her suggestions regarding diet, supplements and lifestyle changes saved me from feeling like death. I want people to understand the power of this way of eating. If you are feeling miserable and not getting the answers you are seeking from your doctors, why not give this plan a try? — Kathy K."

Health tip to try today: try eating PFVx3

In the beginning, I recommend eating three meals a day that include protein, fat and vegetables. For now, focus on adding in these foods intentionally. If you normally just eat a salad with a squeeze of fresh lemon for lunch, then include three or four ounces of chicken or fish to the salad and add olive oil to the fresh lemon juice as dressing. At dinner, aim for two servings of vegetables with a serving of meat, fish or chicken and add butter or coconut oil to your vegetables.

Eating vegetables three times a day seems difficult at first, but will soon be an enjoyable, healthy-building habit.

CHAPTER 12

BEGINNING THE PLAN IS LIKE
BOWLING WITH BUMPERS

My mission is to help you learn how to be as healthy as you can be and to keep it as simple as possible. It can be simple, even though we are all different and there really is no one-size-fits-all diet plan. We differ in age, gender, genetics, digestive health, chronic health conditions, stress levels, cooking abilities, available time and financial resources.

We need structure in the beginning.

Over the years, I have found that in the beginning most people need a specific plan, a list of foods to eat, a timeframe, and recommendations that work for a variety of lifestyles. I like to give plenty of guidance to help you have success during your first few weeks transitioning to this way of eating.

Our parents didn't point to a shiny new two-wheeler in the garage and say, "That's all you need, kid. You will figure it out. Hop on and ride." No, our parents gave us some pointers and ran alongside as we learned to ride the bike. When we start a new job, typically an experienced person shows us how to do the job. We follow their direction because they can shorten the learning curve for us.

Following a trusted mentor is always comforting when wading into new and unknown waters. I will lay out the plan in the next chapter, and I will run alongside you too if you choose to join my facebook community, Whole Healthy Journey.

It is like bowling with bumpers. I will set up the bumpers so that you will be able to stay in the lane and enjoy success from following the plan. The fastest way to begin feeling your best is to follow an eating plan that has consistently worked for others. I am your mentor and I am here to help you. I am a nutritionist, and I have been guiding people into better health for nearly 20 years.

I have a simple plan that works if you follow it. I ask that you commit to being "all in" for one month and you will be astounded with the results. If you are used to eating more processed food than real food, that is the typical starting point for many people. The good news is that you can quickly change course.

I have helped scores of people just like you abandon their failing Standard American Diet. Usually, once they have a grasp on the plan and go shopping, they are off and running in as little as one day. Their dedication and tenacity seems to correlate with how miserable they feel and how badly they want to get better.

If you have been adding more anti-inflammatory foods from the list in Part 2, while reducing the processed foods in your diet, you are heading in the right direction.

In Part 4, I will share the details of the Reclaim Diet Plan and how to eliminate common foods that are causing inflammatory reactions for many people.

Choose the day you will begin the Reclaim Diet Plan.

For me, the choice was clear. I wanted to do something to get rid of chronic hives, and I followed a trusted mentor. I decided to begin as soon as I understood the plan. I ate what was recommended and I didn't stray because my goal was to get better as fast as possible.

You can decide when you will start. Maybe it is not tomorrow, but look at your calendar and pick a day that you will begin the plan. It is fine to begin slowly making changes. You might feel more comfortable changing one meal at a time. At some point though, you will have the best results when you make the switch 100% onto Phase 1 of the plan. Phase 1, the elimination diet, is a 30-day commitment to diligently following these guidelines.

Mark the day that you will draw a line in the sand and let go of processed and allergenic foods for one month. Let this idea grow within you, even if you are the only person in your household willing to make this change. Be all in for 30 days, and your life will change!

Melissa Foster's story is a powerful reminder that many chronic health conditions have inflammation as an underlying cause. Ditching inflammatory foods was life-changing for Melissa and her family.

The Fosters saw their health slipping away and their medications mounting.

Melissa, age 52, was going through menopause and experiencing tremendous hot flashes. She had several health concerns including hypothyroidism, extra weight, vertigo and pain. Her energy was low and she dealt with plantar fasciitis and brain fog. Vertigo led to panic issues. Melissa had a lot of pain due to osteoarthritis. Her knee pain was severe and she needed to use a cane to assist walking.

Doctors prescribed synthetic hormones for her sluggish thyroid and hot flashes, but these did not work well for her. She was also given prescription medications for Dysautonomia (a Central Nervous System issue) and Ménière's disease, but she continued to feel worse and worse.

While researching anti-inflammatory diets, Melissa stumbled upon my website, GetBetterWellness.com, and joined our Facebook group, Whole Healthy Journey. She followed my recommended eating plan and began to have positive results fairly quickly.

"Within 10 days, I realized my knee wasn't hurting." Knowing the level of pain she was experiencing, Melissa said she wouldn't have believed that changing her diet would give her these dramatic improvements in such a short time. "I could see the swelling had reduced in the knee."

Once Melissa felt her pain and inflammation reducing she began to see that her clothes were fitting better. She went on to lose 37 pounds.

Melissa found better support for her thyroid using desiccated thyroid medication instead of the synthetic Synthroid initially prescribed for her. For menopause symptoms, Melissa started using essential oils after watching my YouTube class about Happy Hormones. She got off the synthetic hormones and found that bioidentical progesterone, in an essential oil serum, was what her body needed.

Melissa continues to make beneficial lifestyle choices for her own health and that of her family. She feels empowered to use real food, supplements and essential oils to bring her body to its optimum level.

"I still have to work at eating clean but it has gotten easier and it helps that my husband and adult children still at home are onboard also. I can now wear clothes I haven't been able to wear in years. My husband, a type 2 diabetic, lost 20 pounds and dropped his Hemoglobin A1C from nine to six in about three months! Thanks again for all you do for those looking to live healthier. It was really a blessing to find you!" — Melissa Foster

In the previous chapter, I shared with you 10 benefits you can enjoy when you eat real food and how important it is to eat protein, fat and vegetables for each of three meals a day. This real food eating plan will help you move away from processed food, toward a nutrient-rich, natural, wholesome diet. This shift will help stop the intake of hundreds of chemicals, dyes, additives and preservatives that food manufacturers put in processed food.

Health is rapidly declining in people of all ages. Trends show Americans spend more of their grocery money on processed foods and less on meat and produce than we did in the past. Keeping in step with the increased consumption of processed foods is the rise in obesity, diabetes and chronic illness. When we kick processed food to the curb and give our body whole foods, amazing things begin to happen.

As people begin to think about what changes need to be made, the questions start popping up. Let's address the common questions around processed food, grains, beans and dairy.

Health tip to try today: Choose the day you will start the 30-day, Phase 1 elimination diet.

The details will be given in Part 4, but go ahead and look at your calendar now and choose your starting date. If you are going on vacation or getting married, plan around your big events!

Chapter 13

(FAQs) Common Questions You Might Have As You Begin

Question: What is processed food?

Typically, processed food comes from a factory and real food comes from a farm.

Processed food is often sold in boxes, cans, plastic packages, aseptic containers and jars. Processed food has a label showing ingredients. Real food doesn't need a label. It has one ingredient, and it is perishable. In a grocery store, you can find real food in the produce department and around the perimeter of the store. There are some packaged foods that I recommend, like canned salmon or nuts and certain condiments. I will give tips on how to choose wisely.

"When it comes to our health, especially the health of our children, we are in the eleventh hour. We are seeing the consequences of three generations of processed food displacing the nutrient-dense foods of our ancestors. The good news is that there is still time to turn things around with a [traditional] diet." — Sally Fallon Morell, WiseTraditions.org

Build your diet around unprocessed foods.

We focus on eating traditional, natural foods to achieve optimal health.

The bulk of the diet is based on eating:

- Quality animal foods (beef, pork, venison, bison, poultry, seafood, organ meats, eggs and bone broth).
- Healthy fats (butter, lard, tallow, olive oil, avocado oil, coconut oil, macadamia nut oil, nuts, seeds, olives, coconut, and avocado).
- Colorful vegetables at every meal.
- Some fruit can tuck in here and there. It is best eaten as a dessert following a meal containing protein, fat and vegetables. As a snack, fruit can be paired with a healthy fat/protein to keep your blood sugar stable (apple with almond butter, berries with coconut milk, tangerine with a handful of nuts). Eating fruit without fat/protein is not recommended because it will not be as satiating, it will increase your blood sugar too fast, and leave you wanting more carbs.

Question: What about grains and legumes?

Grains and legumes are not recommended. This is often surprising to many people because our government and most doctors and dietitians have been telling us to eat more grains and legumes. I will list some of the problems with these foods to help you understand why they are problematic today and how they have contributed to people being overweight and sick.

For those with autoimmune conditions, these foods need to remain out of the diet. If you do not have autoimmune conditions, you might be able to include small amounts of organic, properly prepared, gluten-free grains and legumes back in your diet during Phase 3 and Phase 4. I will explain more in the next few sections that may lead you to conclude that all grains and legumes may be best left on the store shelves.

Three health-damaging reasons to avoid grains and legumes

1. High carbohydrates

2. Antinutrients

3. Contamination with pesticides and herbicides

Most of us grew up believing that eating grains and beans was health-promoting. We trusted the authorities but their advice was wrong. If you are tired of being sick, you have to seek truth and be willing to change when given compelling information that contradicts long-held beliefs.

1. High carbohydrates

Grains and legumes and the processed foods containing them are typically high in carbohydrates, promoting weight gain, insulin resistance and high insulin levels.

Cutting out grains and legumes helps you move toward reducing carbohydrates in your diet. Instead of getting your carbs from grains and legumes, enjoy eating a diet rich in other plants (vegetables, fruit, seeds, nuts). Eating this way improves health dramatically (39).

- Reduces blood sugar and insulin (the fat-storage hormone)
- Increases weight loss, if needed
- Decrease belly fat
- Improves cholesterol and triglyceride levels

Cool beans and not cool beans!

Isn't it confusing that the word "beans" is attached to so many different foods and so many phrases? There's green beans, coffee beans, vanilla beans, cocoa beans, kidney beans, black beans and red beans. A ball can hit you on the bean, you can be full of beans and maybe you don't know beans about computers.

When it comes to sorting beans we can think about cool beans (coffee, vanilla, cacao) and not cool beans (soybeans, peanuts, kidney beans, black beans, pinto beans, navy beans, pea protein), and then there are those middle-of-the-road beans (chickpeas, green peas, lentils, green beans).

Legumes are mostly starch and only a little protein. For many people, they are not easily digested because they have a certain kind of fiber that can cause digestive issues, like gas and bloating. Dried beans like kidney, black, pinto and navy are very starchy.

One cup of kidney beans has 40 grams of carbohydrate, a hefty amount. If you are trying to lose weight or keep your blood sugar levels stable, "not cool beans" are off the menu.

2. Antinutrients

Antinutrients are chemicals found in certain plants that bind vitamins and minerals and prevent your body from absorbing nutrients. Some of the health problems caused by eating too many antinutrients include inflammation, digestive issues and brain fog.

While there are certain steps you can take (soaking, sprouting, fermenting) to reduce the negative effects of antinutrients, most people do not have the expertise or the time required to properly prepare grains and legumes, so avoidance is best. Here are the top four antinutrients and why they may be problematic.

- Phytates (phytic acid)
- Lectins
- Oxalates
- Gluten

Phytates (phytic acid) in grains and legumes bind minerals like iron, zinc, magnesium and calcium. Instead of your body getting the benefit of the minerals from your food, phytic acid is carrying them out of the body. Mineral deficiencies and bone loss can result. Phytates are toxic to the body's cells, immune system, and brain. Some of the highest phytate levels are found in soybeans.

Lectin is a protein that can damage the gut and cause bloating, gas and indigestion. Lectins in grains and legumes irritate the lining of the intestine and pass through the gut wall into the bloodstream causing inflammation and damage to other organs and cells in the body. Lectins aggravate autoimmune conditions and damage the cardiovascular system and the brain (40).

Oxalates occur naturally in most plants. Oxalates are normally broken down by healthy bacteria in our digestive tract. For those who have a compromised gut (from poor diet, gut infections, toxins, antibiotic use, stress, food allergies) this normal breakdown of oxalates may not be happening. When oxalates enter the bloodstream instead of being excreted from the body, crystals can form, causing pain and inflammation.

Foods highest in oxalates per serving include rice, buckwheat, rhubarb, wheat, corn, soy, navy beans, almonds, spinach, beets, beet greens. Minimizing the amount of foods high in oxalates may help improve joint pain, signs of aging and autoimmune conditions (41).

Gluten is the protein typically found in wheat, barley, rye, kamut and spelt, and it contaminates oats. The wheat we eat today is not the wheat of the Bible. Humans have manipulated the genetics of the wheat plant so that wheat has 50% more gluten than it did 50 years ago. It is ubiquitous in the food supply and is found in many processed foods including bread, pasta, beer, soy sauce, crackers, condiments and baked goods.

Gluten is hard to digest and it irritates and inflames the digestive system. Gluten is a common source of allergies and sensitivities. Gluten causes leaky gut, a condition that allows partially digested food to escape out of the digestive tract and into the bloodstream. The immune system is triggered by these food particles setting off a cascade of events that can lead to inflammation throughout the body, including your thyroid, brain, skin, heart and gut.

Are you experiencing joint pain, hives and rashes, autoimmune diseases, thyroid issues, diarrhea or constipation, chronic fatigue, acid reflux, brain fog or stubborn weight gain? It is possible that you have leaky gut and the first step in healing is to remove foods that damage the gut (like grains and legumes) and replace those foods with healthy, healing foods.

Is there a way to avoid antinutrients?

Soaking and sprouting grains, seeds and nuts will increase the ability to digest the food and absorb more nutrients, but it does not completely remove all antinutrients.

Lectin is the main antinutrient in legumes. Lectins are broken down by heat. If you soak dried beans in water with salt for 12 to 24 hours, rinse, drain and then cook them for three hours, the lectins and phytic acid are broken down and inactivated but they can still be difficult to digest. It may not be worth your time and effort to eat the "not cool beans" when you consider that the nutrients in beans can easily be found in other foods (without worry). Lentils are often contaminated with small stones and barley (gluten). All lentils need to be cleaned and sorted carefully. Those who strictly avoid gluten may not want to risk a cross contamination of lentils with barley. Lentils need to be soaked for 10-12 hours, rinsed and cooked. Soaking and cooking removes 76% of the phytic acid.

Canned beans and canned lentils have not been properly prepared by soaking and cooking, so it is best to avoid them.

For the first 30 days on the Reclaim Diet plan, I do not recommend eating any legumes, including lentils. This will allow time for your digestive system to heal. In Phase 3 or Phase 4, if you want to try properly prepared legumes in moderate portions, a few times a week, that is an option. Just be sure to buy organic dried beans to avoid contamination with glyphosate (Roundup®). You can read more about that in section three of this chapter.

Soy has problems that go beyond antinutrients

Soy causes more health problems than other beans. Like all legumes it has antinutrients that are not easily destroyed by cooking. There are four other reasons to never consume soy, unless it is small amounts of organic, fermented soy (miso, natto, tempeh).

- Soy contains goitrogens that inhibit thyroid function.
- Currently, 94-percent of soy in the United States is genetically modified. Genetically modified organisms (GMOs) are not safe to eat. Organic soybean fields have been cross-contaminated with genetically modified soybeans.

- Soy has phytoestrogens that mimic estrogen in the human body. This contributes to cancer, reproductive problems, and abnormal sexual development in infants (42).
- Infants fed soy formula receive the estrogen equivalent of at least five birth control pills per day (43).

If you would like to learn more about soy, I wrote an article called, *Soybean in the Crossfire.* You can find it on my website, GetBetterWellness.com.

Why I recommend avoiding peanuts

Peanuts are legumes with quite a few special problems. I recommend avoiding peanuts, peanut butter and peanut oil. Peanuts are high in lectins and they are often contaminated with aflatoxin, a mold toxin. Aflatoxin is known to cause liver cancer (44). The contamination happens in the field and in storage, and is found in both conventional and organic peanuts.

Peanuts grow underground, so they readily concentrate pesticides, fungicides and herbicides from the ground. The USDA Pesticide Program found several pesticides in peanut butter. Many health experts are starting to wonder if the surge in peanut allergies has more to do with aflatoxin and the toxic chemicals sprayed on peanuts than the peanut itself.

3. Contamination of grains and legumes with pesticides and herbicides

Even if you can handle the excess carbs in grains and beans and you properly prepare them by soaking and sprouting to remove antinutrients, we have another evil to consider. This could be one of the biggest reasons to avoid grains and legumes—the presence of pesticides and herbicides, like glyphosate. Glyphosate is the active ingredient in Monsanto's weedkiller, Roundup®. The problems go way beyond the cancer it causes, but let's start there.

Roundup kills human cells. More than 50,000 plaintiffs have now filed suit against Monsanto (a subsidiary of Bayer), claiming their non-Hodgkin's lymphoma was directly caused by exposure to Roundup. In the initial court cases, the jury awarded in excess of $2 billion to people diagnosed with this cancer due to Roundup. "The lawsuits additionally allege that the company was well aware of the dangers but did nothing to warn consumers, working instead to manipulate the scientific record (45)."

It is unlikely that many Roundup cancer cases will be heard in the courts as Bayer seeks to end litigation and sweep this health disaster away with a global settlement.

Maybe you personally do not use Roundup at home, but most people are exposed from food. The chemical-based agriculture system is responsible for poisoning our food supply. Monsanto has genetically engineered seeds so that when the plant grows, the field can be doused with Roundup and only the weeds die. These seeds are called "Roundup Ready" and include soy, corn, canola, cotton, sugar (from sugar beets), alfalfa and sorghum (the latter two are used for livestock feed).

Grains and legumes contain Roundup® residue (sometimes even organic)

Grains (like wheat, barley, oats) and legumes are sprayed with Roundup shortly before harvest to kill the plants so they dry out and can get to market faster. Significant residue remains on the plant and because some organic grains and beans have been shown to contain glyphosate, we know that they are being contaminated somewhere in the process.

The Detox Project tested eight top-selling pea protein powders and found glyphosate in five of the eight powders. What was even more shocking is that the highest levels of the herbicide were found in organic brands. Direct use of Roundup is prohibited in organic foods, yet it was present. Besides direct application, grains and legumes could have been contaminated by glyphosate drifts from neighboring farms, or contamination can happen in a facility that handles organic and non-organic legumes and grains.

Does the government protect you from eating Roundup®?

The EPA sets specific limits on the level of glyphosate residue that can remain in our food and WHO sets the acceptable daily intake (ADI) for glyphosate. This is absurd that there are "acceptable daily intake" levels set for poisonous herbicides. I just want to eat food without Roundup, and I do not agree that there is any ADI when it comes to labeling food as safe for human and animal consumption.

If you eat processed foods with grains and legumes, you are eating Roundup®

Processed food is loaded with Roundup-contaminated corn, soy, wheat, sugar, pea protein and oats. Studies found the herbicide in pizza, flour, crackers, pasta, oat-based products, cereal, food bars and soy-based foods (46).

Glyphosate is absorbed into the plants, and it cannot be removed by washing, baking or cooking the grains and legumes.

Eating weedkiller in grains and legumes can damage health

Dr. Stephanie Seneff, Senior Research Scientist at MIT, regularly speaks, writes and researches the topic of glyphosate and its impact on health.

Dr. Seneff has published many scientific papers and reports that this weedkiller can (47):

- affect the kidneys
- go into the testes and cause damage that leads to cancers
- disrupt the cells that protect the sperm
- paralyze the gut
- contribute to obesity and depression
- mess with the liver

Other studies (46, 48) have shown that glyphosate:

- kills healthy gut bacteria but not pathogenic forms
- disrupts hormones
- impacts the immune system
- promotes inflammation
- opens the door to pathogens like *H. pylori* (connected to ulcers)
- binds with minerals in our body, making them unusable
- damages the powerhouse of our cells (mitochondria)

Remind me why I don't want to eat grains and legumes?

Grains and legumes are not recommended for these top reasons:

1.   High carbohydrates in grains and legumes raise your blood sugar too high. Regular consumption of grains, legumes and processed foods that contain them leads to chronically high insulin levels. This can set the stage for being overweight and having metabolic diseases like diabetes, heart disease and high blood pressure (49).

2.   Antinutrients bind vitamins and minerals and prevent your body from absorbing nutrients. Inflammation, digestive issues and brain fog may result. Soaking, sprouting and long cooking times may address some of the antinutrients, but most people are not sourcing organic grains and legumes and are not properly preparing them so that they are digestible. Gluten cannot be removed from wheat, barley, rye, kamut and spelt.

3.   Pesticide and herbicide contamination has detrimental effects on health and has been found in organic grains and legumes.

Question: Why is dairy being eliminated in the plan?

Most people react poorly to dairy. Removing dairy can clear up skin rashes, including eczema, rosacea and acne. Dairy often causes sinus issues, asthma, allergies, reflux, congestion and digestive issues. Dairy is not a food recommended for people with leaky gut, autoimmune conditions or gluten sensitivity. People who react to gluten tend to also react to dairy.

The commercial dairy industry pasteurizes and homogenizes milk from cows that are given hormones and antibiotics and typically fed an unnatural diet. The cow's feed may contain genetically modified ingredients and may be laced with herbicides and pesticides. The milk that is on the store shelves today is considered the most allergenic food in America.

A distinction needs to be made between raw dairy from grass-fed cows and commercial dairy from conventionally raised cows.

Jonathan R. Kerr, professor of epidemiology, Universidad del Rosario, Bogota, Colombia, wrote, "Whole raw milk, from grass-fed cows, is an enhanced source of nutrients, including beneficial bacteria such as *Lactobacillus acidophilus* and high levels of vitamins (A, B, C, D, E, K), enzymes, calcium, conjugated linoleic acid, in a package that optimizes absorption of all its contents.

Pasteurization reduces contamination with pathogens but also kills the beneficial lactobacilli that produce vitamin K2, improve absorption of nutrients, and normalize gut function (50)."

Pasteurized dairy may be causing your excess mucus, sinus and respiratory problems, rashes, acne, constipation, diarrhea, bloating and gas. Time to say goodbye to those issues!

In Part 4, you will have all the details to begin Phase 1 of the Reclaim Diet Plan, which includes eliminating certain foods known to trigger inflammation and immune reactions for many people. Part of this plan is to remove all dairy from your diet for 30 days, including ice cream, cheese, yogurt and cream. Think about the various places you might find added dairy, and if you are unsure, it is best to avoid the food. Creamy soups, sauces, cheesy casseroles, chocolate, whey protein powder, pudding and custard are examples of foods to avoid during the first 30 days. Quality ghee and butter, like Kerrygold or other butter from grass-fed cows, are fine to include, unless you are aware of a specific intolerance to butter.

So many people believe that they have no problem with gluten and dairy, and I still challenge them to prove it to themselves by removing those foods for 30 days. You might be like Tracie who was able to reverse many chronic health conditions and lose over 50 pounds by following this plan.

Tracie found out that dairy was holding her back from clear skin and weight loss.

Tracie discovered that dairy was one of the foods holding her back from experiencing optimal health and weight. Tracie and her husband attended a class I taught at their church. While they made some progress initially, it wasn't until they decided to be "all in" and follow the plan fully that they experienced dramatic results, losing a combined 91 pounds!

Tracie and her husband were both overweight but had several other medical problems between the two of them including acid reflux, heartburn, digestive complaints, lack of energy, rosacea, and insulin-dependent diabetes. They decided to follow my recommended real food plan fully and try a new way of eating. They focused on eating healthy fats, protein, veggies and only a small amount of fruit, mostly berries. They removed gluten, grains, processed food, sugar and dairy from their diet.

After almost six months of following this plan, Tracie said, "We are experiencing significant positive results. My rosacea has cleared up dramatically and I no longer need to control it with prescription medication. My husband has been taken off of insulin shots! His doctor feels that as long as he stays on this plan, he will be able to remain off insulin."

After 10 months, Tracie reported, "I am down 51 pounds and my husband is down 40 pounds! No more heartburn and the rosacea cleared up tremendously.

I have so much more mental clarity and energy. I no longer have slumps during the day where I feel like I need a nap. My self confidence has increased. I no longer avoid having my picture taken. Thanks for all your help and encouragement. I still want to lose more weight, but even when I get there, this is the new life for me. I don't want to be fat again." — Tracie Reynolds

CHAPTER 14
CAN VEGAN AND VEGETARIAN DIETS BE A HEALTHY OPTION?

Christians often wonder if it is healthier to be a vegan, since God gave Adam and Even the Garden of Eden with edible plants. They probably did not eat meat, even though animals were also there, but it is not clear. God does not dictate how we all must eat, but it is clear that animals were allowed for food:

- After the flood, God said to Noah and his sons, "Every living creature will be food for you; as I gave the green plants, I have given you everything." (Genesis 9).

- Later, God provided quail for the Israelites in the desert. (Exodus 16).

- Jesus fed the multitudes with fish, and he ate it himself after His resurrection (Matthew 14-15, John 21)

- God spoke to Peter and said eat the four-footed animals, wild beasts, reptiles and birds. (Acts 11)

- God created animals, and he cares for their well-being. He cares more for the well-being of humans than animals. (Psalms 104, Matthew 10)

Biblically, it is not wrong to eat meat, nor are we commanded to eat meat. Regardless of your concern for the Biblical narrative, next we need to consider the benefits and drawbacks of eating a vegan or vegetarian diet. The idea is noble: save the planet, save the animals, and improve your health.

Factory farming is wrong and horrible for animals, humans and the environment, but we have access to animal foods from animals raised sustainably that are healthy for humans and the earth.

The experiment of eating vegan has failed people time and time again.

Most people who try the vegan diet do not last three months because they feel poorly and eventually their body takes over and drives the person to eat animal protein. We cannot get all of our required nutrients exclusively from plants. Plant-based diets *can* be nutritionally adequate with supplementation—but not everyone understands what is needed and many people do not take supplements.

"Vegetarian, and especially vegan, diets are lower in several essential nutrients, including vitamins A, B12, and D, as well as calcium, iron, zinc, iodine, choline, selenium, creatine, taurine, methionine, glycine, and EPA and DHA. This is especially true if bioavailability— the portion of a nutrient that is absorbed in the digestive tract—is considered. Studies suggest that vegetarians and vegans are significantly more likely to be deficient in these nutrients (51)."

Veganism is unsuitable for children and may not be healthy for the brain. There are several brain nutrients that are not in plants: creatine, carnosine, taurine, EPA, DHA, B12, D3 and heme iron. "There are so many unknowns," says Nathan Cofnas, who authored a review study on veganism. "And when you deviate from the typical diet for your species, to one which has not been tested and properly established to be healthy or good for the brain, you are conducting an experiment and you are taking a risk." (52, 53)

A plant-based diet can be healthy by including supplements, grass-fed raw dairy, eggs and fish regularly along with vegetables, fruit, seeds and nuts (ovo-lacto-pescatarian).

I appreciate that you may have ethical reasons for avoiding animal foods. I am completely against factory farming for the catastrophic environmental impact and concerns for animal welfare. When animals are raised on feedlots and fed an unnatural diet (including organic feed), we get cheap food at a high cost—pollution, animal abuse, unnecessary hormones and antibiotics, and inferior food quality. It is impossible to be a vegan and not hurt animals when you are eating plant foods like soy, grains and legumes that come from industrial farming operations. The destruction of the land harms all life, including animals, insects, birds and soil microbes.

"Every day there is a new confirmation of how destructive, inefficient, wasteful, cruel and unhealthy the industrial agriculture machine is.

We need a total rethink of our food and farming systems before it's too late." — Philip Lymbery, chief executive of Compassion in World Farming (54)

A plant-based diet is not the answer to factory farming and it is not the optimal diet for most humans. Grassfed, pasture-raised and free-range animal products and wild-caught fish are raised sustainably and provide nutrients we need. There will be far greater impact on the environment when meat-eaters seek sustainably raised animal foods compared to the fraction of a percent of vegans abstaining from meat. All life is valuable, especially human life. Before choosing to live life as a vegan, carefully consider the health challenges that you may face.

Health challenges reported by former vegans

Remember Alexandra Jamieson, the "vegan girlfriend" and co-creator of Super Size Me? She started eating a vegan diet as a way to reboot her body, suffering from years of unhealthy eating. It was a great cleanse and she felt better for a while, but then there was a shift. She became chronically anemic, developed hypothyroidism and insomnia and felt depressed and exhausted. She tried for a year to do everything within the vegan realm to overcome these health challenges, to no avail. Her body was craving meat, fish and eggs but Alexandra didn't want to contribute to animals' suffering. "I began to realize that we need to offer compassion for all creatures, all animals, all humans, ourselves, in order to be truly compassionate. I believe you can love and care about animal welfare and still consume them."

Angelina Jolie, actress. "I joke that a big juicy steak is my beauty secret," said Jolie. "But seriously, I love red meat. I was a vegan for a long time, and it nearly killed me. I found I was not getting enough nutrition."

Anne Hathaway, actress. A long-time vegan, Hathaway was in Iceland and she was served fresh wild salmon. As a vegan, she did not feel good or healthy or strong. "So I had a piece of salmon and my brain felt like a computer rebooting," she said.

Yovana Mendoza Ayres, aka Rawvana, 6-year vegan. When Yovana initially went vegan, she felt great. After about one year, she stopped getting her period and was anemic. She began to feel tired and was diagnosed with candida overgrowth. She cut the fruit and grains to overcome the condition, but developed SIBO (small intestinal bacterial overgrowth). Yovana decided to add animal products into her diet to recover.

Tim Sheiff, former plant-based athlete. Tim added animal foods back in his diet after feeling stiff every morning. He noticed that his joints were creaking and he felt "desperate for health."

Lierre Keith, author and 20-year vegan. "I started when I was 16 and as you might guess my health failed catastrophically." At age 18, two years after being a vegan her spine started to fall apart and she developed degenerative disc disease. She stopped menstruating, which is very common among women who are either vegan or eat low-fat diets. She over consumed soy and wheat and developed an autoimmune disease and had abnormal blood sugar levels. Lierre, like a lot of vegans, had dry skin, dry hair, and extreme exhaustion. She felt freezing cold all the time and developed depression and anxiety. After 20 years, she gave up her vegan lifestyle and began eating animal foods. Most of her health issues resolved, some immediately, but other issues seem to be permanent. To read her story, get the book, *The Vegetarian Myth.*

I advocate that people eat moderate amounts of clean animal protein, plenty of colorful vegetables and healthy fat with smaller amounts of fruit, seeds and nuts. Eating this way covers your nutrient bases without having to know about nutrients.

Health tip to try today: Meal planning

Changing dietary habits will be much easier with a little planning. Before you begin the 30-day elimination diet, practice planning meals for the next three days. Remember to include protein, added fat (butter, coconut oil, avocado oil, olive oil, olives, avocados) and a few servings of vegetables at every meal. If the grocery store is not too far away, you may find it easier to shop twice a week while you are learning how much protein and fresh produce to have on hand.

CHAPTER 15

THREE WAYS TO SHIFT YOUR MINDSET AND EMBRACE CHANGE THAT HEALS

In the previous chapter, we covered the common questions people typically have as they prepare for this healing journey. Before we get into the actual plan, let's talk about how to have a healthy mindset.

1. Renew your thinking—you are not on a diet!

The fastest way to feeling your best is to avoid thinking like a dieter. Dieters think about how hungry they are on their deprivation diets and they talk about having a "cheat day" or "being on a diet/off a diet" and "being bad" or eating bad food.

Food is not your enemy. Food—real food—is a gift. There are so many delicious treats and healthy options that we can enjoy to replace unhealthy foods.

I encourage you to renew your thinking and begin to see yourself as someone who deserves to feel amazing and look great. You are making a commitment to your health by upgrading your food choices and creating a new lifestyle.

Of course, I want you to be "all in" during the 30-day elimination diet, but if you don't follow the plan to the letter, it does not mean you failed and need to go eat a pan of brownies. I want you to learn how to listen to the cues that your body is giving you so that you can adjust and find the path that is right for you.

If you are ready to renew your thinking, here's a tip: hide the scale. The scale can sabotage your feelings about your progress. If you tend to weigh yourself regularly, you know how discouraging that practice can be. Hide the scale and and change your thoughts. The scale is a poor indicator of healing. It is better to focus on how good you feel, how your clothes are fitting, how much energy you have, how much better you sleep and how much you love eating real food.

2. Change the chatter in your head

"Never affirm or repeat about your health what you do not wish to be true." – Ralph Waldo Trine

We all have an internal dialogue in our head. For some, it is like a tape that keeps playing, telling a story that may not be true. Many people have a tape that plays inside their mind that says, "You can't do this, you always fail." Or maybe you are hearing yourself say, "This is too hard! Who can live without bread and cheese?"

While I know that this eating plan will help you heal and lose weight fast without feeling deprived and miserable, you will enjoy greater success when you change the internal thoughts to be positive and supportive. This time you WILL be successful.

Terri Savelle Foy, teaches about learning the language of success through positive declarations in her book, *Pep Talk*. Terri wrote,

"The first step to improvement is becoming conscious of what you are saying in your mind about yourself and to yourself.

"The instant you find yourself affirming negative statements and behaviors about yourself, STOP! Instead of using your words to describe how you feel, use your words to change how you feel."

Instead of saying, "No matter what I do, I can't lose weight." STOP and say, "I am grateful that choosing real food increases my metabolism."

Instead of saying, "I can't stop eating bread and cheese." STOP and say, "I am free from food and bondage to food."

Instead of saying, "I have tried before, and nothing works." STOP and say, "I am healing my body and I am enjoying the process of being in the best shape of my life."

Write out a list of positive declarations that you can read when the negative thoughts start creeping in. Make your list personal and as long as it needs to be to combat every negative thought. Here's a start:

- I love eating real food.
- I am disciplined and full of energy.
- I enjoy being healthy and working out.

3. The 30-day elimination diet (Phase 1) is the fastest way to heal and break food addictions

The Reclaim Diet plan works and it will work for you. After a few transition steps, it begins with an elimination diet to check for food sensitivities. You will eat delicious, whole food while you eliminate certain foods from your diet. The elimination diet is only 30 days. Following this time-limited plan will bring you into a new place where food cravings and food addictions no longer drive your eating behavior.

I am not a fan of "intuitive eating" during these first few months of healing. Intuitive eating is an idea that humans can simply listen to their body's cues and eat without restrictions of any kind of food. Most people are reacting to ingredients in processed food, wheat and commercial dairy. These problem foods and the presence of certain infections (like candidiasis) can create enormous cravings for foods that will fan the flames of inflammation and illness.

You will discover that the free recipe book I have for you in the Facebook group, Whole Healthy Journey, will give you a variety of nourishing, delicious meals and snacks. Be sure to pop over to the group and request to be added.

Health tip to try today: Write down positive declarations.

Write out a list of positive declarations that you can read when the negative thoughts start creeping in.

PART IV

THE RECLAIM DIET PLAN TO GET YOUR LIFE BACK

Part 4 will give the details of the four-phase Reclaim Diet plan. You will learn when to eat, what to eat and how to make wise choices when shopping for food. The four phases of the Reclaim Diet are powerful and will help you identify specific foods causing or contributing to health concerns. At the same time, you will flood your body with nutrient-rich foods and connect with food as it was for our ancestors—pure, simple and nourishing.

Imagine how much better you will feel as you shift away from poor eating patterns that create a downward spiral leading to poor health. You will begin to feel empowered as you explore a commonsense approach to eating. If you have had an adversarial relationship with food in the past, you will connect with the wholesome goodness of real food. This book is not about giving you a rigid set of rules. Rather, it guides you back to a place where you can reclaim control and power over your health so that you can build from the ground up.

Transitioning to a healthier way of eating is different for everyone. Some people just want to start feeling better as fast as possible and will jump right into compliantly following Phase 1, the elimination diet (Chapter 20). The downside of making an abrupt, dramatic change is that it may be hard on your body and for those who are not already preparing meals without the use of processed food, it can feel like you spend a huge amount of time cooking food and washing dishes. On a positive note, if you are not feeling well, and need big health changes, jumping in as fast as possible will get you closer to your goal in the shortest amount of time.

It is your choice whether you choose to transition abruptly or more slowly. Either way, let me provide you with a quick overview and a step-by-step guide to help you start incorporating healthy foods today.

CHAPTER 16

BUILD YOUR CONFIDENCE WITH A COUPLE OF BABY STEPS

The goal of the Reclaim Diet is to eliminate as much refined and processed food as possible and focus on eating meals with clean animal protein, healthy fats and nutrient-rich vegetables, fruits, seeds and nuts. Let's build a healthy diet from the ground up. Follow these simple steps to begin incorporating nourishing foods into your day and then move into Phase 1, the 30-day elimination diet.

Step 1: Eat three meals daily, and one snack between meals

Step 2: Transition breakfast to real food

Step 3: Transition lunch to real food

Step 4: Transition dinner to real food

Step 5: Transition between-meal snacks to real food

Step 6: The 30-day elimination diet (Phase 1)

Step 7: Reintroduce foods after the 30-day elimination diet (Phase 2)

Step 8: Customize your own real food plan (Phase 3)

Step 9: Move forward on your healthy journey (Phase 4)

Step 1

The first baby step, without any requirements around *what* you are eating, pay attention to *when* you are eating. Plan three meals a day, and limit snacks to one snack between meals, without grazing and constant nibbling. Having breakfast at 6:00 a.m. and then skipping lunch will make you ravenous later in the day. You will be extremely hungry and start gobbling down any food you can get your hands on. Skipping meals is not only unpleasant but it causes the body to feel stress. The stressful feeling can trigger the adrenal glands to release the stress hormone, cortisol. Cortisol can trigger inflammation and the storage of belly fat and unwanted weight gain.

Eventually, most people do not feel the need for a snack once they are eating PFV meals. Either way, avoid grazing and snacking your way through the day to give your body a chance to burn body fat instead of storing it. Americans tend to eat every few hours, grazing all day long. Let's stop that bad habit and dispel the notion that humans need to eat six or more times a day. Studies have shown that there is no advantage to eating frequent, small meals (55). In fact, eating more frequently is associated with increased likelihood of overweight and central obesity (the big belly associated with diabetes and heart disease) (56).

After a few days focusing on when you are eating, it is time to pay attention to what you are eating.

Step 2

Transition breakfast to real food first. Eating protein, fat and vegetables at breakfast (PFV) will keep your blood sugar balanced and steady in the morning. Now it is time to transition your first meal to include PFV.

If you have not been a breakfast eater, you can train yourself to enjoy a nourishing meal before you start your day. Remember that a cup of coffee and a gluten-free KIND® Bar is not a PFV breakfast. Why? The bar is processed, lacks quality animal protein, and it is high in carbohydrates (often from sugar, honey and grains). You will get a spike in your blood sugar but when that spike drops, it leaves you hungry and looking for another snack. A KIND® Bar might be an acceptable occasional snack later on, but for the first 30 days, we are eating unprocessed, real food three times a day.

The next few chapters provide all the details for choosing quality animal protein, healthy fat and carbs from vegetables, fruit, seeds and nuts. For now you can plan some simple real food meals for breakfast with a vegetable omelet cooked in butter or olive oil and a side organic sausage. You might even like having left over chicken with broccoli and peppers, sauteed in healthy fat like avocado oil or olive oil. If you enjoy fruit, add berries or a small serving of other fruit. Avoid eating processed foods, baked goods and grains for breakfast during this transition. After a few days you will feel good about planning and eating a PFV breakfast.

Step 3

Transition lunch to real food next. While you continue to eat a PFV breakfast, now incorporate protein, fat and vegetables for lunch. This might be a salad with 3 or 4 ounces of meat, fish or chicken and an olive oil and vinegar dressing or a beef burger, without the bun, and a side salad with avocado, red onion, and tomatoes. Once you have been eating a PFV breakfast and lunch for at least three or four days, turn your attention to making dinner nutrient-rich.

Step 4

Transition dinner to real food. Continue to eat a PFV breakfast and lunch and now plan a few real food dinners. Animal protein with two vegetables will be a good goal. For example, try chicken stir-fry with vegetables, seasoned with coconut aminos or have broiled fish with steamed broccoli and sweet potatoes, topped with butter. Skip the pasta and bread at dinner.

Step 5

If you are eating snacks between meals, transition to a real-food snack when you are hungry. Nutrient rich snacks include protein and fat if possible. Eventually, as your metabolism heals, you will not be hungry for the snack. Eating too often causes a hormone problem called leptin resistance, with weight gain and uncontrollable cravings for food. Byron Richards, author of *The Leptin Diet*, wrote, "Snacking is the primary cause of inefficient metabolism leading to obesity and the early onset of disease."

Real food snacks can be a cup of leftover egg salad with carrot sticks for dipping, or guacamole and vegetables or a small apple sliced and dipped in a tablespoon of almond butter.

Now we will talk about what to eat and how to make quality choices when shopping for food.

CHAPTER 17

QUALITY ANIMAL PROTEIN

Fish, chicken, meat and eggs are the best sources of all the essential amino acids that your body requires. This plan is considered a moderate protein diet. It is not a high protein diet, which can be hard on the body. Moderate protein is about three or four ounces of meat, fish or chicken per meal (that's about 20-30 grams of protein per meal). Having just one egg will not give you adequate protein, since one egg only has about 7 grams of protein. Instead, it is better to eat two or three eggs with some breakfast sausage and veggies cooked in butter or coconut oil.

Most people need 60 to 90 grams of protein per day. To determine how much protein you require, use the following calculation: Ideal body weight in pounds (what you would like to weigh as a perfectly healthy, lean person) divided by 2.2 = your weight in kilograms (kg). Daily, consume 1.2 to 1.7 grams of protein per kilogram of body weight. Divide your daily protein intake among three meals. Pregnant women, athletes and men typically need a little more protein.

There is an online calculator to help determine your ideal body weight in kilograms. Visit ClinCalc.com and look for the "Ideal Body Weight Calculator."

Some people, especially older adults, have trouble digesting animal protein. If you experience frequent bloating, nausea, constipation, bad breath, body odor or feel sluggish after eating, you may not be properly digesting protein. The key is to supplement with digestive enzymes and betaine HCl capsules at meals containing protein. These supplements help with the breakdown of protein so that the body can utilize the nutrients efficiently.

Here are the benefits you will enjoy by including animal protein in your meals:

- provides all nine essential amino acids required by the body
- functions as building blocks for the body's framework, skin, hair, nails, muscles, organs and ligaments
- keeps blood sugar levels stable
- reduces carbohydrate cravings
- spikes energy levels and increases fat metabolism
- increases satiety and sustains muscle during weight loss
- favorably influences metabolic rate to benefit weight loss efforts
- provides amino acids from which the body makes the happy brain chemicals called neurotransmitters
- strengthens the immune system, providing adequate zinc and protein to make antibodies
- provides raw materials for the body to make hormones and enzymes

- transports oxygen to the body's tissues as hemoglobin, the iron-containing protein in red blood cells
- provides a higher quality, more digestible source of protein over plant protein

Examples of healthy animal protein

(Ideally from grass-fed, free-range, wild-caught, pasture-raised sources):

Meat	Poultry	Seafood	Shellfish
Beef	Chicken	Salmon	Shrimp
Pork	Turkey	Cod	Scallop
Venison	Goose	Trout	Lobster
Lamb	Quail	Herring	Oysters
Elk	Pheasant	Mackerel	Mussels
Bison	Duck	Sardines	Crab
Rabbit	Poultry eggs	Trout	Clams

Meat consumer tips:

Big business meat production operations raise animals in a way that is not good for them, for us or the environment. These concentrated animal feeding operations (CAFOs) confine the animals in crowded and unsanitary spaces, feed them an unnatural diet and pump them full of growth-promoters, hormones, and antibiotics.

A report posted on the Centers for Disease Control and Prevention (CDC) website stated that manure from CAFOs is a major health issue because of the amount of manure produced. One large feeding operation with 800,000 pigs can produce 1.6 million tons of manure a year. The manure contains pathogens like *E. coli*, growth hormones, antibiotics, and excess nutrients like nitrogen and phosphorus. There is runoff and leaching into the groundwater, contaminating the area, the water and sometimes the crops grown nearby.

The goal of a CAFO is to grow animals faster, bigger and cheaper. That means finding the cheapest food possible, including genetically modified corn and soy and mixing the feed with chicken manure and feathers, bakery waste (bread, donuts) and unsellable candy like Skittles, gummy worms and chocolate bars.

The healthiest meats are from wild game or sustainably raised, 100% grass-fed and grass-finished animals. These animals are treated humanely, eat a natural diet, get fresh air and have space to roam and graze. Their meat is healthy and has a higher content of vitamins, minerals, antioxidants and good fats—omega-3s and CLA—than CAFO meat. We will talk more about omega-3 fatty acids in the section on healthy fats, but eating pasture-raised meat will provide more omega-3s which protect against heart disease and inflammation.

If the thought of finding a small family farm seems daunting and beyond your budget, check out the resources below.

Here are a few tips to fit quality meats into your budget:

1. Buy in bulk from local farmers. This may mean that you are buying 1/8 or 1/4 share of an animal. It will be divided and packaged for you. Buying all cuts of beef in bulk will only cost you an overall average price of $4 to $6 per pound, including steaks!

2. Ground meat is always the most affordable. Again, if you can buy in bulk, you may be able to get pasture-raised ground meat for $2 to $3 per pound.

3. Learn ways to stretch meat by cooking stews and soups loaded with vegetables.

4. Try experimenting with cheaper cuts and organ meat from grass-fed beef, bison or lamb.

5. Buy from reputable online sources like US Wellness Meats and WallaceFarms.com.

6. Chicken thighs and chicken with the skin on are healthy options. Chicken skin is high in monounsaturated fat (like olive oil and avocados). Plus, cooking chicken with the skin on helps retain flavor and moisture.

You do not need to be 100% perfect when it comes to sourcing quality food, but I want you to be 100% aware that it absolutely matters how our food is raised, and we vote with our dollars. As more people become aware of the drawbacks of CAFOs and seek better options, we can begin to effect change in the system.

Resources:

EatWild.com

EatWellGuide.org

Poultry consumer tips:

When buying poultry look for pastured (pasture-raised) poultry first. Pastured poultry describes a method of farming chickens, turkeys, ducks, geese, guineas and eggs.

Certified organic is a marketing label from the USDA, but it does not require that the poultry is pasture-raised. In fact, 90% of certified organic poultry on the market does not come from animals raised outdoors on fresh vegetation.

Conventional chicken farming production is different from pastured poultry (chickens raised in as natural an environment as possible). Pastured poultry is raised outdoors in fresh air, with daily rotation of the pens, to provide fresh green vegetation and bugs. Chickens consume vegetation and insects, and their manure helps build soils. The birds get exercise and eat a natural diet which imparts more flavor to the meat. A roasted pastured bird is not only healthier, but it is more meaty and juicier than a conventionally raised bird.

Seek local, small flock poultry producers who are raising birds on pasture. While supplementing the diet is often necessary, birds given a soy-free diet will have a healthier ratio of omega-6 to omega-3 fatty acids (57).

Learn more:

"Pastured Poultry: Better Way Forward" video:

https://youtu.be/PdLnF5jQcXg

Check out this pastured poultry buying guide to find pastured chicken, eggs, turkey, ducks, geese and more near you:

https://apppa.org/Directory

Fish and seafood consumer tips:

In general, when purchasing seafood look for wild-caught fish instead of farm-raised fish. Most grocery stores will sell wild-caught fish in the frozen food section. You will also find canned wild-caught salmon, tuna and sardines.

Farmed Fish vs Wild-Caught Fish

The nutritional value of farmed raised fish depends on their diet and how they are raised. Farmed salmon, for example, may be fed a diet that includes corn, wheat, soy, fish meal pellets, poultry byproducts, fish oil, and vegetable oil (like soy and canola). Salmon fed this diet will have a higher fat content, with visible white lines of fat. The ratio of omega-3 fats to omega-6 fats is altered, with wild-caught salmon having a favorable ratio of fats compared to farmed salmon. Farmed salmon have a higher amount of the inflammatory omega-6 fats and wild salmon has higher amounts of beneficial omega-3 fats.

Farmed salmon are grey in color and are given natural or synthetic pigment to create the desirable pink color. Synthetic pigments are created from petrochemicals.

Farmed salmon are raised in net pens, often in crowded conditions. They are susceptible to more infections from bacteria and parasites including sea lice. Sick fish are treated with antibiotics and other chemicals.

To be fair, not all farm-raised salmon are the same. The Norwegian aquaculture industry sets a higher standard for sustainably farmed salmon than countries like Chile. Norwegian salmon are fed an all-natural diet, and the salmon's pink color comes from a natural carotenoid, astaxanthin. The pens allow more freedom and great care is taken to keep the ecosystem in balance. If wild-caught salmon is not available, I would trust sustainably raised salmon from Norway or New Zealand.

To learn more about sustainably raised fish, visit the website SeaFoodWatch.org. Their recommendations show you which seafood items are "Best Choices" or "Good Alternatives" and which ones you should "Avoid."

When purchasing fish, the package will indicate the country of origin. Avoid seafood from Asian countries, including China, Vietnam, India, Indonesia and Thailand. A common practice in Asia is to raise fish and seafood on pig feces and waste from poultry. Shrimp farmed in Asia often involves the heavy use of antibiotics and chemicals to keep shrimp alive in crowded pens. Look for shrimp from the U.S., Nova Scotia, and Canada.

What about mercury in seafood?

While some ocean fish are contaminated with mercury, the concern that we are "eating mercury" when we eat fish is offset by the selenium content of the fish.

Oceans are rich in selenium, and selenium acts like a "mercury magnet" as long as the fish has more selenium than mercury. Studies show that swordfish and pilot whale are two types of fish to avoid since the ratio of selenium to mercury is not favorable (58).

While the "mercury magnet" ratio helps, this does not give us liberty to consume tuna with abandon. I do not recommend eating tuna more than two or three times a week, especially when consuming tuna caught from deep ocean waters. There are reports and published case studies of people over-consuming tuna and experiencing ill effects. One 48-year-old man was experiencing pain, tingling, burning and numbness in both legs, and his condition was deteriorating. For two months, he was tested and treated for an unknown musculoskeletal disease. Finally, he was asked about his occupation. For 15 years the man worked on a tuna fishing vessel, spending one year at sea at a time. While on board for one year, the man consumed tuna twice a day, almost every day (over one pound a day). His blood mercury levels were tested and he was diagnosed with mercury poisoning (59).

The mercury content of tuna rises with the age and size of the fish. The best tuna is from sources using only pole and line as well as troll-caught tuna. These smaller, younger fish caught closer to the surface of the water have lower levels of mercury compared to the older, larger tuna caught at much lower depths of the ocean.

Companies like Wild Planet and Vital Choice use these sustainable catch methods and have proven, via third party testing, to have significantly lower levels of mercury than many national companies (60).

Omega-3 content of seafood

Omega-3 fatty acids are important essential fats. Essential means the body cannot make it and we must consume these essential fats in our diet. Omega-3 fatty acids are known to fight inflammation and cardiovascular disease and promote eye and brain health. We can get omega-3 fats from the meat and organs of grass-fed meats, wild game and wild-caught cold-water fish. I also recommend supplementing omega-3 from fish oil or cod liver oil.

Fish ranked by beneficial omega-3 fatty acid content:

Best (>500 mg omega-3 per 3.5 oz serving)

- Salmon
- Herring
- Mackerel
- Sardines
- Trout
- Anchovies
- Canned albacore tuna
- Canned Wild Alaskan Salmon
- Arctic char
- Oysters
- Mussels

Good (150 - 500 mg of omega-3 per 3.5 oz serving)

- Haddock
- Cod
- Halibut
- Shrimp
- Sole
- Flounder
- Perch
- Alaskan King Crab
- Pollock
- Rockfish

- Clams
- Crab
- Lobster
- Snapper
- Grouper

Low (<150 mg of omega-3 per 3.5 oz serving)

- Mahi Mahi
- Red snapper
- Grouper
- Tuna, wild
- Scallops
- Shrimp

Poor, little to no omega-3

- Tilapia
- Farmed catfish

Health tip to try today: Take some time to review the resources mentioned in this chapter and begin to find local farmers and stores that offer quality animal protein. If you use Facebook, check for local real food communities that can recommend real food providers.

CHAPTER 18

HEALTHY FAT

Healthy fat is not the "baddie" of all nutrients. Contrary to the commonly held belief that fat is bad and makes you sick and overweight, healthy fat is critical for optimal health and is responsible for a huge list of health benefits.

The French Paradox

The French apparently do everything wrong (according to conventional thinking) and yet their incidence of cardiovascular disease and stroke is low. Their diet has always been rich in saturated fat (61). Some wonder if it is the wine that is helping the French stay healthy. Instead of trying to pinpoint one simple explanation for the French Paradox, it is better to consider their diet as a whole along with their lifestyle.

Observations regarding habits of the French: (62)

- Ninety-percent of French adults eat a diverse diet, compared to 33% in the US.
- They drink wine (60% of French women drink one glass or less per day).
- They consume fresh, seasonal foods and 30% of the homes have gardens.
- Eating is a pleasurable, social experience.

The French enjoy better health because of their diet. It is not a paradox.

The French are not afraid of healthy fat, or rich nutrient-dense foods.

They regularly serve red meat, butter, cheese and organ meat at meals.

School lunches in France reflect their values.

The journal, *Childhood Obesity*, published an article by Jodi Godfrey about the school lunch program in France, "French children willingly eat everything that they are offered, and most of what they are offered is healthy." Children in the public school system are given freshly prepared three- and four-course hot lunches. School, governments and communities work together to educate families and create systems to feed children well (63).

To learn more about how parents can learn from the French model and raise happy, healthy eaters, pick up a copy of Karen LeBillon's book, *French Kids Eat Everything*.

"You'll sometimes hear about the 'French paradox', which describes the phenomenon of low heart disease rates in France 'despite' a diet rich in saturated fat. Well, it seems that this 'paradox' is not limited to France, but is alive and well in several other countries too, including the U.K., Germany, Austria, Finland, Belgium, Iceland, the Netherlands and Switzerland.

"In other words, it's not a paradox at all. It's only a paradox if one believes saturated fat causes heart disease. The thing is, there's really no good evidence that it does." — Dr. John Briffa, integrative medicine physician and top graduate of the University College London School of Medicine.

We Must Eat Quality, Healthy Fats

To lose weight and enjoy optimal health, we must eat healthy fats, ideally at every meal and snack. Eating fat does not make you fat. It is not unusual to find people avoiding natural fat, and eating low-fat and fat-free food. This misguided thinking comes from years of hearing that "fat is bad" and causes heart disease, high cholesterol and excess weight gain. For the last 40 years, so-called experts have promoted the notion that butter, meat and eggs must be avoided while we were told to use "heart healthy" oils like canola, soy, sunflower, safflower, corn and peanut oil. These oils actually create inflammation and contribute to heart disease and other chronic health conditions.

Fat Deficiency

Americans are following the anti-fat recommendations, yet heart disease is growing, obesity is skyrocketing, chronic diseases and infertility are rampant.

Do you deal with any of these symptoms of fat deficiency?

- Constantly hungry
- Have cravings for fried food, ice cream and sweets
- Feel fatigued, and often have a mid-afternoon energy drop
- Blood sugar lows or highs

- Unable to lose weight
- Dry skin and dry eyes
- Skin rashes
- Unhealthy looking skin with rough, bumpy and dry areas, wrinkles
- Hormonal imbalances
- Digestive problems (IBS, gas, bloating)
- Gallbladder ailments
- Hypothyroidism, thyroid imbalance
- Dry, brittle hair and nails
- Difficulty with focus and cognition
- Mood swings, depression, anxiety
- Infections (bacterial, fungal, viral)

If you are not consuming healthy fats and use inflammatory, processed oils, you are fat deficient. Seed oils and vegetable oils like sunflower, safflower, corn oil, soy oil, and canola oil are highly processed. The food industry uses damaging processes in order to extract oil from seeds, corn, peanuts and soy. Often the oils are extracted from genetically modified plants (corn, soy, canola) that have been treated with Roundup® and other harsh chemicals. Extreme heat and chemicals, like hexane, are used to extract the oil. The process leaves a stinky, damaged oil that must be steamed and deodorized before it can be sold.

Processed vegetable and seed oils (even cold-pressed and expeller-pressed) are high in omega-6 fats which increase inflammation in the body and in the arteries. These oils interfere with healthy cellular function, lower your immune system and even impair brain function.

Processed foods (baked goods, crackers, chips, candy bars, frozen meals, fake whipped cream) are loaded with inflammatory oils because they give the product a longer shelf life. Restaurants typically use cheaper oils to save money and rarely use healthy fats and oils to prepare food (french fries, fried chicken, salad dressings, sauces, dips, oils for cooking and baking).

Avoid or limit the following oils and products:

Corn Oil	Sunflower Oil	Smart Balance	Margarine
Canola Oil	Safflower Oil	I Can't Believe It's Not Butter	Spreadable Butter with Canola Oil
Grapeseed Oil	Peanut Oil	Country Crock, Buttery Spread	Earth Balance
Soybean Oil	Cottonseed Oil	Any Vegetable Oil Spread	Light Butter with Canola
Vegetable Oil	Palm Kernel Oil	Any "Plant Butter"	Move Over Butter

Enjoy Eating Healthy Fats Daily

Good fats heal and provide a variety of health benefits shown below. Include healthy natural fat in every meal and snack.

Add about 1 Tbsp of fat per meal, or roughly 10 - 12 grams. Added healthy fat may come from extra-virgin olive oil (EVOO) in salad dressing, or butter added to cooked vegetables. Cook with healthy fats and intentionally add foods like avocado and olives.

Quality matters, as always, especially with fats. Extra-virgin olive oil will ideally list the country of origin and the date the oil was produced. Extra-virgin olive oil is the least processed and will have more health benefits than virgin olive oil or pure olive oil. Animal fats should come from healthy animals raised properly. This plan incorporates plenty of healthy fats, oils and animal foods.

Healthy fat benefits:

- helps with weight loss
- provides a concentrated source of energy without raising blood sugar or insulin
- helps build healthy cell membranes so that cells can take nutrients in and get toxins out efficiently
- supports the hormonal system and fertility
- transports cholesterol to the tissues where it is used in cellular repair and needed to make hormones
- slows the absorption of nutrients so we feel full longer
- helps with the absorption of fat-soluble vitamins: A, E, D, K

- helps us have healthier skin and hair
- supports brain health (sharper brain, clearer thinking)
- supports bone health and helps calcium get into bones
- helps protect your heart and raise the heart-protective HDL cholesterol
- carries micronutrients throughout the body
- supports a healthy digestive system

Examples of Healthy Fats for Cooking

Low to High Heat Cooking	Low to Moderate Heat Cooking
Ghee, organic	Butter, grass-fed
Extra-virgin olive oil	
Avocado oil	
Coconut oil	
Macadamia nut oil	
Algae oil	
Red palm oil from the fruit (Nutiva) Avoid palm kernel oil from the seed.	
Duck fat, lard, tallow (only if rendered from wild or pasture-raised animals)	

Examples of Foods Containing Healthy Fats:

Olives, cured (no vinegar)	Grass-fed meat
Avocado, guacamole	Wild-caught fatty fish
Coconut, coconut milk	Free-range eggs
Nuts (about ¼ cup, 1-2 times a day)	Fish oil
	MCT oil

Coconut Oil is a Superstar

Incorporate unrefined coconut oil into your diet. This is a major player in enhancing energy and weight loss. It is unlike any other oil due to its chemical structure. It is metabolized in the liver and used right away as energy.

You can use it for a stir fry, or for baking vegetables and sweet potato fries. Try cooking eggs in coconut oil or add 1 Tbsp to smoothies or a cup of hot tea.

Unrefined coconut oil benefits: (64)

- raises metabolism and helps with weight loss
- makes you lean because it creates energy and is not stored as fat
- has antibacterial, antifungal, antiviral properties due to the fatty acid, lauric acid, also found in mother's milk
- lessens the effect of PMS and menopause
- stabilizes the blood sugar and is one of the best oils for diabetics
- acts as a great moisturizer for the skin
- very stable when heated
- easier to digest for those without a gallbladder

Be sure to visit the CoconutResearchCenter.org to read personal testimonies from people using coconut oil and experiencing a multitude of health benefits.

Life-Changing Omega-3 Fatty Acids

I recommend consuming omega-3 fatty acids in the form of food or supplements to avoid a deficiency. They have incredible health benefits documented in the scientific literature: (65, 66, 67)

- reduce inflammation, which may help lower heart disease, cancer and arthritis
- improve insulin sensitivity so that the body needs less insulin to help the cells absorb glucose from the blood
- help regulate the nervous system, blood pressure and blood sugar
- provide beneficial effects for asthma
- reduce joint stiffness and pain
- enhance recovery and optimize training gains in athletes
- reduce the risk of illness
- improve brain function
- fight depression (68)
- improve eye health (69)
- improve cardiovascular health (70)
- provide benefits for skin health (71)

We all want those benefits, right? Just be sure to regularly consume wild-caught fish and pasture-raised animal foods. These sources have beneficial long-chain omega-3 fats, EPA and DHA. Plant foods like flax, hemp and walnuts have short-chain omega-3 fats.

The body is not very efficient at taking the plant-based omega-3s (ALA) and converting them into what it prefers, EPA and DHA. Less than 8% of plant-based omega-3s actually get converted to EPA and less than 1.0% of ALA is converted to DHA (72).

Most of the health benefits provided by omega-3s come from the animal form, the longer chain fats, EPA and DHA. Be sure to eat plenty of wild-caught fish and free-range animal foods. It is a good idea to supplement with a high quality omega-3 supplement that provides about 1,000 mg of DHA.

Health tip to try today: Do you need an "oil change"? Review the list of unhealthy oils and check your pantry. Replace unhealthy oils with quality fats and incorporate them intentionally into your meals.

CHAPTER 19

CHOICE CARBOHYDRATES

There are a wide variety of opinions on how carbohydrates fit into a healthy diet. Should we eat low carb, high carb, no carb, vegetarian, vegan, grain-free, sugar-free, potato-chip-free, high popcorn, no popcorn, low glycemic, ten-bananas-a-day diet, the cookie diet, or how about the fruitarian diet?

The last three, unfortunately, are real fad diets that people follow. Eating only fruit or cookies will not lead to long-term vibrant health and, as I mentioned earlier, neither will a vegan diet.

The types of carbs that are the most nutrient-dense are vegetables, fruit, seeds and nuts. Previously I shared why grains and legumes are problematic carbohydrate foods, so let's now look at some recommendations for including vegetables, fruit, seeds and nuts.

There is no one-size-fits-all when it comes to how many carbs are best. I always recommend that people take one month and eat a nutrient-dense, lower carbohydrate way by following a plan that is grain-free, dairy-free and free of processed food. The best way to discover which foods are causing a reaction in you is to complete an elimination diet (Phase 1). I will share more about the elimination diet in the next chapter. The foundation of this healing eating plan is to build meals around quality animal protein, healthy fat and mostly vegetable carbohydrates.Eating a low-carb, nutrient rich diet is the fastest way to fix metabolism and blood sugar imbalances. It is important to recognize that all carbohydrate foods turn into sugar (glucose) and raise your insulin levels, but non-starchy vegetables have very few carbohydrates and are not a concern.

The average American consumes too many added sugars (technically, caloric sweeteners). When reading the ingredients' label on packaged food it is sometimes tricky to spot these sugars, but they include white table sugar, rice syrup, dextrose, barley malt, corn syrup, agave nectar, Florida crystals, coconut sugar and more than 50 other sweeteners. The annual consumption has been reported to be as high as 158 pounds of added sweeteners for the average American adult and more for kids. It is not hard to believe that people are consuming a cup of added sweeteners each day when we consider that various sugars are added to processed food, including candy, cakes, bread, bagels, soup, cereal, peanut butter, ketchup, mayonnaise, salad dressing, baked goods, coffee drinks, juice, sport drinks, soda, and more.

The government has decided that Americans need to keep added sugars to no more than 10% of the diet. What does that mean? Will Americans read packages, and calculate how many calories of added sugars they are eating? Will people ask the fast food restaurant or gas station how many added sugars are in their meal or Slurpee? There is no way to follow the government's recommendation unless you stop eating processed food. Even then, it is a bad idea to allow 10% of your daily calories to come from sugar. That is about 12 to 15 teaspoons a day for the average person. The amount of added sweeteners we need is zero. When eating a low-carb, real food plan, there can be fun treats (visit GetBetterWellness.com for healthy dessert recipes) and sometimes you may choose to add a little raw honey or other less refined sweetener to coffee or tea, but on a daily basis you will not want to get anywhere close to 15 teaspoons a day.

Cancer cells are sugar addicts.

This is a powerful statement and is the title of an article written by:

Ellen Davis, first published in *Well Being Journal,* September/October 2013.

"As good as sugar may taste, IT IS NOT YOUR FRIEND! It's the friend of cancer, heart disease, diabetes, weight gain, fatigue, Alzheimer's and focus issues. Plus, it has created a growing health epidemic in our country and around the world, particularly with children. Sugar is big business. And they want you to be addicted."
— Jonathan Otto, Get Off Your Sugar Summit

Many people tell me, "I don't really eat sugar." I am not just referring to the white stuff in the sugar bowl, or the chocolate chip cookies and ice cream. We all know sugar is in these foods. Sugar (glucose) mostly comes from carbohydrates that we eat. The "Ten Bananas a Day Diet" is not only nutritionally insufficient, but ten bananas equal 300 grams of carbs and convert into 75 teaspoons (about 1.5 cups) of sugar (glucose). This much glucose is taxing on the body and is likely to end up as stored fat. A half a banana would be a reasonable serving of fruit. Here's a chart to show you the carbohydrate content of fruit and how many teaspoons of sugar that a serving size becomes in your bloodstream. This information is to show you that you can enjoy most fruit, but as the carbohydrates increase, be aware that it is best to reduce the portion size.

I recommend limiting fruit to 0 to 3 servings per day. Enjoy fruit as a dessert after a meal or pair it with protein and/or fat (a tangerine and a handful of nuts, an apple with a tablespoon of almond butter or a grass-fed beef stick with a kiwi).

Fruit	Serving Size	Carbohydrates, grams	Tsp of Sugar (glucose)	Notes
Lemon/lime	1 small	6	1.5	
Tangerine	1 small	9	2.25	
Kiwi	1 whole	10	2.5	
Fig, fresh	1 medium	10	2.5	
Strawberries	1 cup	12	3.0	
Coconut	1 cup	12	3.0	
Cranberries	1 cup	12	3.0	
Blackberries	1 cup	14	4.7	
Raspberries	1 cup	15	3.75	
Peach	1 medium	15	3.75	
Cantaloupe	1 cup of balls	15	3.75	
Orange	1 medium	18	4.5	
Apple	1 medium	20	5	reduce to 1/2 apple per serving
Cherries	1 cup	20	5	reduce to 1/2 cup per serving
Blueberries	1 cup	20	5	reduce to 1/2 cup per serving
Pineapple	1 cup	22	5.5	reduce to 1/2 cup per serving
Pear	1 medium	26	6.5	reduce to 1/2 pear per serving

Grapefruit	1 medium	26	6.5	reduce to 1/4 or 1/2 grapefruit per serving
Mango	1 cup	28	7	reduce to 1/2 cup per serving
Grapes	1 cup	29	7.25	reduce to 1/2 cup per serving
Banana	1 medium	30	7.5	reduce to 1/2 banana per serving
Pomegranate	1 cup seeds	36	9	reduce to 1/2 cup seeds
Dates	1 cup	133	33.25	Not recommended
Raisins	1 cup	131	32.75	Not recommended

Avoid dried fruit and fruit juice

Dried fruit is concentrated sugar, as you saw in the previous chart, and dried fruit may be contaminated with mold. Fruit juice (even freshly pressed) does not have fiber, which helps slow the absorption of carbohydrates. Shockingly, orange juice has just as many carbs as a can of Coke (39 grams per 12 ounces, which converts to about 10 teaspoons of sugar after consuming). Most juice is pasteurized, damaging the nutrients, while leaving all the carbs. It is best to eat fresh whole fruit so that you get the benefits of the whole food with the fiber.

Six to nine servings of vegetables?

It may seem impossible to eat six to nine servings of vegetables each day. For me, it was overwhelming in the beginning since I was barely eating more than baby carrots and iceberg lettuce! Including a variety of colorful vegetables into your day will give your body a boost of nutrition and you will feel the difference.

Maybe you will feel more comfortable starting with three servings of vegetables a day. Enjoy a colorful salad at lunch and have one or two vegetables at dinner, and then begin to work your way up in baby steps.

The World Health Organization defined a serving of vegetables to be about:

- 1 cup raw vegetables
- 1/2 cup cooked vegetables
- 2 cups raw leafy greens

Terry Wahls, MD, is a physician who reversed her progressive multiple sclerosis by eating a nutrient rich diet. Check out her Tedx Talk, "Minding Your Mitochondria." Dr. Wahls was severely disabled, nearly bedridden, when she turned to nutrition. She learned what nutrients were needed for a healthy brain and nervous system.

"It occurred to me that I should get my long list of nutrients from food [rather than supplements]. That if I did that, I would probably get hundreds and maybe thousands of other compounds that science had yet to name, that would be helpful to my brain and my mitochondria." — Dr. Terry Wahls

Dr. Wahls recommends eating a variety of vegetables each day. Eat one third of your vegetables as leafy greens, one third as deeply colored vegetables (three different colors daily), and one third as sulfur-rich vegetables.

Leafy green vegetables include chard and kale, cilantro and parsley, bitter greens (beet, collard, dandelion, mustard, turnip) and all types of lettuce, except iceberg.

Have some fun in the produce department or at the farmer's market trying to find a variety of colorful vegetables to bring home.

Sulfur-rich vegetables

Sulfur-rich vegetables support the liver and help with the removal of toxins from the body. In her book, *The Wahls Protocol*, Dr. Wahls lists several other known health benefits of consuming sulfur-rich foods:

- anti-cancer properties

- antimicrobial action

- blood vessel health

- gut health

- heart health

- hormone balance

- immune system support

- Here are some sulfur-rich vegetables:

- brussels sprouts

- cabbage

- cauliflower

- garlic

- ginger

- onions, scallions

- broccoli

- broccoli sprouts or microgreens

- radishes

- mushrooms

- leeks

- asparagus

Potatoes and rice

Potatoes and rice are super starchy and will turn into too much sugar in your blood. Have you ever seen those gigantic baking potatoes that Costco sells? I once bought a bag of potatoes for the holidays years ago. The front of the bag's marketing slogan was, "Big Taste - Slimmer Waist." The bag boldly claimed, "Only 110 calories and 45% of the RDA for Vitamin C." High in Vitamin C? Don't get too excited, Skittles makes this claim too. So, I did what any suspicious nutritionist would do. I weighed the potato and it clocked in at 1 pound 3 ounces. Those large potatoes have over 400 calories and dump 23 teaspoons of sugar in your bloodstream (from 92 grams of carbohydrate).

How is that going to slim your waist when most of it gets converted to fat? How is that going to help you manage your blood sugar when God designed us to have just 1 teaspoon floating around at any time. Michael Eades, MD, did all the calculations in his blog post, "A spoonful of sugar" to prove that last point (73).

If you want to have a potato occasionally, here's what I recommend:

- Choose sweet potatoes and red-skinned new potatoes over white baking potatoes.
- Monitor the portion size and eat one-half cup or half of a small potato.
- Eat the potato with a meal containing animal protein, fat and two servings of colorful, low-starch vegetables.
- Top the potato with generous amounts of butter or coconut oil.
- Toppings can include chives, green onion, bacon, and broccoli, but skip the pasteurized cheese.
- Try "faux-tatoes" made from riced cauliflower.

Riced cauliflower is a great substitute for rice when avoiding grains. It is available in the freezer section, or you can make your own with a food processor. To cook cauliflower rice, heat a skillet, add fat. Pour in the desired amount of riced cauliflower and cook for about five minutes. Season with salt and pepper and try adding other herbs. We add chopped tomato and turmeric or cilantro and lime for a different flavor combination. You can even use riced cauliflower to make a low-carb version of mashed potatoes. We buy organic frozen riced cauliflower and mix in almond milk or broth and add butter, garlic or other herbs. It is delicious, and even those who claim to be cauliflower haters will be easily tricked!

Have you been told that you NEED to eat grains to be healthy?

Nearly every cell in the body prefers fat as an energy source. The heart prefers fat for fuel in the form of ketones. The parts of the body that need some carbohydrates (glucose), like the brain and the nerves, will do quite well with a low-carb approach. That is because the glucose required can be supplied by the liver via a process called gluconeogenesis (meaning "new glucose") and is made when needed from protein. For fuel, the brain can use 70% ketones (from fat) and 30% of the fuel comes from glucose—either via the diet or created by the liver (74).

Eating a low-carb program decreases the brain's requirement for glucose. The actual amount of carbs that work best for an individual varies, but it is likely between 30 to 150 grams a day. Remember, we are talking about eating six to nine servings of non-starchy vegetables per day as your main source of carbohydrates and adding smaller amounts of fruit, seeds and nuts (75, 76).

Compared to a low-fat diet, research shows that lower carb, higher fat diets:

- are healthier for the brain (77, 78, 79, 80)
- benefit the cardiovascular system (80, 81, 82, 83, 84, 85)
- reduce fatty liver (86)
- result in more weight loss and less hunger (81, 82, 83, 87, 88, 89, 90, 91)
- burn more calories, helping maintain weight loss over a

longer period of time (low-carb groups lost 2-3 times as much weight as the low-fat groups) (92)

- improve fasting blood sugar levels and insulin sensitivity (80, 81, 93)
- offer therapeutic potential for cancer patients (80)

Neurologist David Perlmutter, MD, wrote: "When it comes to eating 'memory food' there is no better trio of items to fight Alzheimer's and dementia than

1. grass-fed beef

2. avocados

3. coconut oil

This group of high-fat, brain-smart foods are a staple of the *Grain Brain* diet, and should work their way into your weekly meal plan as well."

I recommend eliminating grains and legumes while focusing on vegetables as the main source of carbohydrates along with some fruit, seeds and nuts.

Georgia Ede, MD, listed the health benefits of eating a low-carb diet in her article, "8 Reasons to Try Low Carb for Mental Health" (*Psychology Today*, June 2019):

1. Improve blood glucose control.

The higher your blood sugar (from eating excess carbohydrates), the higher your brain sugar (glucose). High glucose levels are toxic to the brain.

2. Lower blood insulin levels.

A high-carb diet repeatedly causes high insulin levels and can damage insulin receptors that the brain needs to process glucose and turn it into energy. Low-carb diets protect brain cells from energy deficits.

3. Reduce inflammation.

High-carb diets promote inflammation in the body and the brain. Inflammation is a root cause of most degenerative diseases and most psychiatric and neurological diseases.

4. Boost antioxidant defenses.

High-carb diets create more oxidative damage than the body's natural antioxidant molecules can neutralize. Cells in the body and the brain are damaged. A low-carb diet helps improve the body's natural antioxidant capacity.

5. Energize mitochondria.

High-carb diets damage the powerhouse of the cell, the mitochondria. Low-carb diets improve the health of the cell's mitochondria.

6. Stabilize stress hormones and appetite.

A high-carb diet upsets good hormonal balance by creating blood sugar highs and lows. People can experience more anxiety, shakiness, sweating, irritability and have difficulty concentrating. Low-carb diets keep blood sugar levels even, and do not trigger abnormal surges in hormones like adrenaline and cortisol.

7. Rebalance neurotransmitters.

Neurotransmitters, or your happy brain chemicals, are disrupted by a high-carb diet. Eating too many refined carbohydrates promotes inflammation and oxidation, switching the brain into an excited state.

8. Raise BDNF levels (Brain-Derived Neurotrophic Factor).

BDNF helps the brain cope with stress and recover from stressful events. When BDNF levels are high, the brain is resilient.

Health tip to try today: Swap out grain and pasta side dishes and add in another serving of colorful vegetables. Try preparing vegetables using different methods—steam, stir fry, roast—always adding a quality healthy fat to increase nutrient absorption.

CHAPTER 20

PHASE 1

ELIMINATION. THE 30-DAY ELIMINATION DIET

We have talked about many different health topics and now it is time to give you a concise, step-by-step plan to follow for 30 days and beyond. Phase 1: Elimination, the elimination diet is followed by Phase 2: Reintroduction. Following this order is the best way to learn how your body responds to certain foods while giving you plenty of nutrient-rich foods that will be nourishing and healing.

The elimination diet is your ticket out of your long list of health woes and weight issues. I wrote about this briefly in Part 2, and now it is time to help you take action. I assure you that you will have plenty of delicious food to eat!

Everyone I have helped, and I mean everyone who has agreed to follow this plan, has had a great outcome and they actually love eating this way.

Here are comments from some folks who were just completing Phase 1, the elimination diet. These comments were taken, as written, from a survey that they completed. I'll share more comments in Chapter 21.

- *My mood is better, more even, much clearer thinking. I really lost my desire for many of the bad foods.*
- *I don't own a scale but I could tell by how my clothes fit (loosely!) that I lost some weight! Energy lasted all day. Regular bowel movements!*
- *The first week was a bit of a challenge, but once I got the hang of it and organized it went MUCH better. I didn't sleep well the first week, but I'm nearing the end of the 3rd week and feel great. I lost about 10 pounds and I think it was mostly waste!!! YUCK. I am now going to focus on getting some good supplements.*
- *I finally broke my weight stall! Ten pounds, and you know that is not easy for me. I no longer need to drink a pot of coffee to function in the morning. I'm not hungry all day long.*
- *My daily allergies were so much better! I do not have to take daily allergy meds anymore.*
- *I really gained back my self-control and confidence as I took time to continue to put my health first. I had more energy and had more clarity.*
- *Less brain fog, no need for sweets. I lost 8 pounds, a weight I have not seen in 10 years*
- *Mid way through the second week, I realized that when I get out of bed I don't feel like an 80 year old. It was totally amazing. My doctor told me a year ago that I should get into physical therapy based on what I described to her about how I felt in the mornings. Never mentioned a word about nutrition.*

Depending on what you are eating now, there will be an adjustment period but it may not be more than a week or ten days. For me, I was eating a diet high in processed foods, including sweets, bread, chips and fast food. I was motivated to follow the elimination diet that my doctor suggested because I wanted to heal from hives as quickly as possible. The first week was hard for me, and I felt unwell making such a drastic change overnight. If I had reduced the processed food I was eating and increased my consumption of nourishing food for a week or two before I had to be 100% on plan with the elimination diet, my symptoms may have been reduced.

As a nutritionist, I always recommend starting with the elimination diet for one month. Completely removing gluten and other problematic foods like dairy, soy, corn, and processed foods can reduce symptoms quickly and start the healing process.

The elimination diet is considered the "gold standard" when uncovering food sensitivities.

Food allergy testing is unreliable and expensive. Go back and read the story in Part 2 about the 14-year-old girl who was tested for wheat allergies and tested normal. It was not until her mother, working with a nutritionist, put the girl on a strict gluten-free diet that she had complete reversal of her symptoms. The elimination diet is the best way to determine if you are reacting to certain foods.

If you are like me, when I was suffering from chronic hives, panic attacks and Hashimoto's Thyroiditis, I needed answers and wanted relief. The SICKcare system only offered me medication. Pills were not going to help me get to the root of the problem as pills only cover symptoms. You deserve to find out what is the root cause of some of your symptoms so that you can heal. I encourage you to take one month to do this valuable experiment called the elimination diet.

Benefits of the elimination diet

The elimination diet has many benefits. It is cleansing to the body and it helps you identify food sensitivities that may be causing or contributing to chronic conditions and stubborn weight issues.

Benefits of the elimination diet may include:

- better mood
- improved skin
- increased energy
- improved sleep
- balanced hormones
- decreased sugar cravings
- weight loss
- reduced pain

What is the elimination diet in a nutshell?

You will focus on eating whole foods that are not processed or refined.

For one month you will eat mostly vegetables, fruit, meat, eggs, fish, poultry, healthy fats, and seeds and nuts while eliminating the most common inflammatory foods.

I realize that if you are not eating this way currently, it can feel overwhelming to adopt a new diet like this. But, trust me, it's not that difficult. The only thing you will be giving up is lack of sleep, lack of energy, pain and unwanted pounds. You will feel better than you have ever felt. Just give this plan one month and you will be amazed at the difference in your health. Many people begin to see results much faster.

Remove common inflammatory foods (listed below) 100% for one month (the first six will be tested during Phase 2: Reintroduction):

1.   all dairy, whey, casein, lactose (except butter and ghee)

2.   all grains

3.   corn

4.   gluten

5.   peanuts

6.   soy, including soy protein, found in energy bars and protein powders and processed soy foods

7.   legumes

8.   artificial ingredients

9.   sugar, including coconut sugar, sugar cane crystals, cane juice and maltodextrin (some honey is fine, ideally raw and organic)

10.   high-fructose corn syrup

11. artificial sweeteners, including aspartame, Sucralose, Splenda and sugar alcohols (sugar alcohols in "-ol" like xylitol)

12. dyes, preservatives and additives

13. inflammatory oils (soy, corn, canola, safflower, sunflower, cottonseed and peanut)

14. margarine, spreads, trans fats and hydrogenated fats

15. processed food, fast food, refined carbohydrates, including crackers, bread, bagels, chips, popcorn, muffins, baked goods, cereal and oatmeal

16. flavored drinks and teas that list "flavors" on the label (herbal, green and oolong tea are all fine — opt for organic when possible)

17. soda, energy drinks, coffee drinks and fruit juice

18. foods known to have a problem with mold (overly ripe fruit, dried fruit and peanuts)

Choose nourishing foods:

Phase 1 is a commitment to simply eating unprocessed food. While the list of ingredients and foods to avoid seems long, just focus on what you *will* eat, nutrient-rich whole food:

- organic, fresh or frozen vegetables and fruit
- organic, pasture-raised meat and poultry
- wild-caught fish
- organic, pasture-raised poultry eggs

- healthy fat like extra virgin olive oil, olives, avocados, avocado oil, organic or grass-fed butter, unrefined coconut oil, seeds, and nuts
- butter and ghee are fine to keep in the diet
- purified water or spring water instead of tap water

Tight budget or limited access to quality food?

I understand, from working with many people over the past 15 years, your budget may be tight and your local grocery store may not offer organic, wild-caught, pasture-raised and free-range food. Do the best you can! It is always better to eat the ground beef you can find and afford, even if it is not from happy cattle, raised 100% on pasture.

The list of nourishing food, above, gives you the ideal quality of food to include, but I do not want anyone to opt-out of the Reclaim Diet because they cannot buy organic or find wild-caught fish. You can afford to eat real food—don't forget, you will be saving money by not purchasing processed food and fast food. You will be amazed that eating ground beef burgers (no bun!) or baked chicken thighs with a big salad will be more filling for you than a pile of spaghetti and sauce that leaves you inflamed and hungry in an hour.

Tips for Phase 1: Elimination

Now that you understand the foods to focus on eating and the foods to eliminate,   I will share tips and ideas to assist you during Phase 1 and beyond. Let's expand on the topic of what to eat and drink, and talk more specifically about what food to avoid. While this book doesn't address other lifestyle factors, I will touch on a few ways to increase health benefits, in addition to diet.

These recommendations are for the first 30 days, during the Phase 1 elimination diet, and will serve as your foundation for healthy eating beyond the first month.

The Reclaim Diet is a lifestyle, not a typical diet that you start and stop, but a way to help you support your body's ability to heal. You will feel more energetic, sleep better, have clearer skin, have less inflammation and enjoy eating in a way that brings you to higher and higher levels of health and wellness.

What to eat

1.   Eat three meals a day. Eat breakfast, lunch and dinner.

2.   Include quality protein (about three to four ounces for women and a little more for men and athletes) with meals. Look for grass-fed meats, wild-caught fish, and free-range chickens and eggs. Do the best you can when sourcing animal protein while you locate better options and farmers' markets.

3.   Include healthy fats (about 1 tablespoon added fat) with each meal. Use organic, grass-fed butter (Kerrygold, Organic Valley), extra-virgin olive oil, avocado oil and unrefined coconut oil. Enjoy avocados, natural olives, nut butters, nuts and seeds.

4.   Focus on increasing your intake of vegetables and include two servings at every meal. Recall from the previous chapter, that one

serving of vegetables is about one cup of raw vegetables, one-half cup cooked vegetables or two cups of raw leafy greens.

5.   A little bit of fruit is fine to have with a meal or as a dessert or with a protein/fat snack. It is easy to over-consume fruit, which can raise blood sugar and may hinder weight loss. About zero to three servings of whole fruit per day is fine for most people. Skip fruit juice and sugary (and often moldy) dried fruit.

6.   Avoid grains, and food made with grains, including bread, pasta, cereal, crackers, baked goods, bagels and muffins, as these will leave you tired and hungry within a few hours. This includes gluten-free processed foods.

7.   Eat a snack if you are hungry, but try to include a little protein and fat in your snack. Raw vegetables dipped in guacamole can be a portable snack when you look for single-serve containers of guacamole. Celery sticks or apple slices paired with one tablespoon of sunflower butter or almond butter is a delicious and satisfying snack. Check out grass-fed beef and turkey sticks from PaleoValley.com.

8.   Eat real food! Packaged food is loaded with chemicals, industrially processed junk oils, sugar, monosodium glutamate (MSG), dyes and other artificial ingredients that hinder healing and weight loss.

9.   Eliminate any unnecessary supplements. Many vitamins purchased at retail stores contain wheat, dairy, soy, corn, dyes and artificial sweeteners that we are trying to avoid. For a list of basic

supplements that most people need, see Appendix B.

What to drink

1.   Drink water. Every morning begin your day by drinking 20 - 24 ounces of purified, room temperature water upon rising (not tap water). Wait 30 minutes before consuming any food or supplements.

2.   During the day consume water regularly.

3.   Drink about half your body weight in ounces of water (a 150 pound person would drink 75 ounces of water).

4.   Try not to drink during meals because this dilutes stomach acid needed to break down food.

5.   To prepare your digestive system for the meal, you may opt to add two or three teaspoons of raw apple cider vinegar to six ounces of water and consume 30 minutes before meals. This step alone has been shown to be beneficial for reducing blood sugar and blood insulin levels in individuals.

6.   A large majority of Americans are dehydrated. Twenty-percent of Americans drink no water at all and 42% drink two cups or less per day. Water is vital for health and essential to life. We cannot live more than a few days without water. Water plays many important roles in the body, like transporting nutrients to the cells and waste products out of the body. Water regulates body temperature and lubricates joints.

7. Limit coffee to one or two cups per day. Avoid cream and creamers. Canned, whole fat coconut milk or unsweetened almond milk, like Califia Farms, is a good option to replace dairy.

8. Organic green tea and herbal tea can be consumed.

9. Sparkling mineral water without additives (like San Pelligrino in the bottle) is an enjoyable treat. Mineral water can be flavored with fresh lemon and lime or Vitality essential oils and liquid stevia drops. Try adding a few teaspoons of raw apple cider vinegar to sparkling mineral water and enjoy the benefits for blood sugar and insulin levels.

10. Limit alcohol to one or two glasses of wine per week (no beer or hard liquor).

Navigating the grocery store

Earlier you learned how to choose quality animal protein, healthy fat and the best carbohydrates. It is time to go shopping! The following tips will help you obtain healthy food from the grocery store. Shop the perimeter of the store where the fresh food is found. This includes the produce department, meat department, and the coolers for butter and eggs.

The aisles are loaded with processed foods but you will venture into the inner aisles to find healthy fats, olives (just olives, water and salt), nuts and seeds (dry roasted or raw are best), herbs, spices, tea, honey, condiments, canned fish, tomatoes (best in glass) and canned coconut milk.

Grab my Grocery Shopping Guide from the Appendix or download a copy from my Facebook group, Whole Healthy Journey.

How to support the liver and the whole body

Include foods that support the liver and aid in detoxification. When you are ready to transition away from processed food, sweets, grains and dairy, you may want to add in a few key liver lovin' foods intentionally during the first seven days, and beyond, to enhance the benefits of your real food plan. Your liver is your hard-working detox organ and it may need some extra nutritional support.

1. Eat at least one serving of food daily from each of the five groups below:

- The juice of one-half of a lemon, or two to three teaspoons of raw apple cider vinegar, added to a glass of water and consumed at least 30 minutes before breakfast (rinse your mouth after consuming fresh lemon juice or vinegar)
- Cruciferous vegetables (cabbage, cauliflower, broccoli and brussels sprouts)
- Green leafy vegetables and herbs (parsley, kale, watercress, chard, cilantro, beet greens, collard greens, escarole, dandelion greens and mustard greens)
- Liver-healing foods (artichoke, asparagus, beets, celery and dandelion root tea)
- Sulfur-rich foods in addition to the cruciferous vegetables already listed (garlic, ginger, onions, broccoli sprouts, eggs, radishes, mushrooms, leeks and asparagus)

2. Movement (three or four times a week)

Walking, strength training, and mild exercise or burst training can be added, but now is not the time to take on a new, vigorous exercise plan. Focus on your nutrition first and as your body heals and your energy increases, you will know when it is time to increase the intensity.

3. Sleep and relaxation

Try to get seven or eight hours of sleep a night. I gave many tips to help you get a good night's sleep back in Chapter 10.

Recipes to get you started on your Real Food Plan

Breakfast ideas

Do not skip breakfast! If you do not like to cook in the morning, I have a recipe for a make-ahead egg bake below. You can also be out the door quickly in the morning if you make a protein smoothie (diary-free, soy-free). I usually take time the night before to make a smoothie with fat (canned coconut milk or avocado), veggies (greens and other vegetables that your blender can handle) and frozen berries. I often will add Collagen Peptides as a source of easy-to-digest protein.

Meal Replacement Smoothie, 2 servings

- 1 Avocado or 1 can of coconut milk, full fat (Native Forest or Natural Value)

- 2 to 4 scoops of collagen peptides

- 16+ oz water and ice, adjust to be the consistency you prefer

- Optional nutrition boost for smoothies:

- 2 cups green leafy vegetables (kale, chard or romaine)

- 1 cup frozen blueberries and/or strawberries or 1 pear or 1 apple

- 1 - 2 tablespoons ground seeds (flax, raw pumpkin, raw sunflower or hemp)

Baked Breakfast Casserole - make ahead and enjoy during the week

Makes a 9x13 inch pan

- 15 eggs, beaten well
- 1/2 of a very large parsnip shredded, about 2 cups
- 1-2 carrots, shredded, about 1 cup
- 3-4 cups of organic baby spinach, roughly chopped
- 1 cup chopped onion
- 1 bell pepper or 4 mini peppers, chopped
- 1/2 cup coconut milk, canned, full fat
- 4 chicken apple sausages, cut into bite-sized pieces
- salt and pepper to taste

1. Preheat your oven to 350 degrees.

2. Grease a 9x13 pan well with coconut oil or avocado oil.

3.   Cook the sausages, spinach and onion in coconut oil, avocado oil or butter until veggies are tender and sausage is browned.

4.   Beat eggs well, add coconut milk and mix well.

5.   Stir the rest of the vegetables into the sausage and spinach combo, and cook for a minute or two.

6.   Add vegetable mixture to the eggs, mixing well.

7.   Pour egg mixture into a 9x13 pan.

8.   Bake for about 30 minutes or so, checking the middle by inserting a knife to see if it comes out clean to test for doneness.

9.   This casserole can be stored in the refrigerator for a few days, cut into squares for a grab-and-go breakfast.

Lunch and dinner recipes

Teriyaki Salmon

- 1/4 cup olive oil
- 1/4 cup fresh lemon juice
- 1/4 cup coconut aminos (a soy-free, gluten-free sauce to replace soy sauce)
- 1 tsp stone-ground mustard (or other gluten-free prepared mustard)
- 1 tsp dried ginger
- 1/4 tsp garlic powder
- 4 wild-caught salmon filets

1. In a plastic bag, combine the first six ingredients and mix well.

2. Set aside 1/4 cup of marinade in the refrigerator for basting.

3. Add salmon to the bag and place in the refrigerator to marinate for one hour.

4. Remove salmon. Discard marinade.

5. Broil or grill salmon for 4-5 minutes per side.

6. Brush with reserved marinade.

Meatloaf and Oven-Baked Sweet Potato Wedges

- 2 pounds ground beef
- 2 fresh, whole tomatoes, chopped
- 2 eggs
- 1/2 cup each carrot, onion, celery, red pepper
- 3 cloves garlic, pressed
- 1/4 tsp pepper
- 1/8 tsp nutmeg
- 1/4 tsp sage
- 1 tsp sea salt

1. Preheat the oven to 350 degrees.

2. Combine all ingredients.

3. Divide between two loaf pans.

4. Peel and chop sweet potatoes into wedges and coat with oil.

Spread on a baking sheet lined with parchment paper for easy clean up.

5.   Bake meatloaf, uncovered, one hour.

6.   The potatoes can go in the oven at the same time.

Crock Pot Beef Stew

Put the following in your crock pot:

- 1 onion, quartered, or about 2 cups of pearl onions, peeled
- 4 carrots, chopped into two-inch pieces
- 2 sweet potatoes, peeled and diced
- 2 ribs celery, cut in chunks
- 4 cloves garlic, minced
- 3 pounds beef stew meat
- 1 tsp Italian seasoning or 1 tsp thyme
- 1 tsp Real Salt or other mineral salt
- 1/8 tsp pepper
- 1/2 tsp garlic powder
- 2 cups gluten-free beef broth

1.   Heat coconut oil or avocado oil in a skillet over high heat and brown the beef cubes on all sides, about one minute per side.

2.   Put all ingredients in the crock pot except the meat and stir.

3.   Add the browned beef, season beef with salt and pepper.

4.   Cover.

5.   Cook on low for 6 to 8 hours.

Cilantro Chicken Quick Stir Fry

- 1 pound chicken, cut into strips

- 1/4 cup avocado or olive oil

- 1 cup cilantro leaves, chopped

- 4 cloves garlic, pressed or finely chopped

- 1 Tbsp ginger, peeled and finely chopped

- 2 onions, thinly sliced

- 1 bell pepper, cut in chunks

- 2 cups broccoli florets, cut into in smaller pieces

- 1 cup sliced mushrooms

- 1 Tbsp lime juice

- Salt and pepper

- 1 Tbsp fresh lemon juice per serving

1.   Mix garlic, ginger, half of the cilantro and the 1/4 cup oil in a bowl.

2.   Add the chicken and put in the refrigerator to marinate for an hour.

3.   Heat a large skillet and stir-fry the chicken.

4.   Remove the chicken to another bowl.

5.   Add additional avocado oil or coconut oil to the skillet and stir fry onion for three minutes.

6.   Add the bell pepper and stir-fry for three more minutes.

7.   Add Broccoli, mushrooms and stir fry for two minutes.

8.   Return chicken to skillet. Add the lime juice and remaining cilantro leaves and cook to heat through and blend the ingredients.

Salads

- Use a variety of greens: romaine, green leaf, red leaf, Boston, mixed greens, and spinach. Skip the anemic iceberg lettuce.
- Make the salad interesting by adding a variety of other ingredients:

1.   Cucumbers, squash, radishes, carrots, fennel, celery, mushrooms, beets, olives or avocado.

2.   Add nuts, such as walnuts, sliced almonds or pecans.

3.   Add seeds, such as sunflower, pumpkin or ground flaxseeds.

4.   Add salmon, tuna, turkey, chicken, eggs or sardines. If this is a main-dish salad, aim for three or four ounces of protein.

5.   Mix in grated carrots, beets and jicama, or add sprouts to the top.

Make your own salad dressing to avoid low-quality ingredients and inflammatory oils typically used in commercial dressing. Some stores will carry two brands of salad dressing that contain good ingredients: Bragg's and Primal Kitchen.

Italian Dressing

- 1 cup olive oil
- ½ cup vinegar, balsamic
- 2 pressed garlic cloves
- ½ tsp dried oregano
- ¼ tsp dried basil
- ¼ tsp onion powder
- ¼ tsp sea salt

Store in a glass shaker bottle

Tuna Salad, Egg Salad, Sardine Salad

When preparing a salad spread, it is important to use a mayonnaise with healthy fat. Look at the ingredients on the label and try to find a product that uses coconut oil, avocado oil or olive oil.

Chicken Salad

- 2 pounds chicken breast, cooked and cubed
- 3 hard boiled eggs
- 1/2 cup apple (with peel, chopped)
- 1-1/2 cups mayonnaise
- 1–½ cups celery, chopped
- 1/2 cup red onion, chopped

- 1 tablespoon lemon juice
- 1/2 - 1 tsp Real Salt or other mineral salt
- 1/4 tsp garlic powder
- 1/2 cup pecans, chopped (optional)

1. Mix all ingredients in a large bowl.

2. Serve chicken salad on a bed of greens.

Makes 6 servings.

Snacks

- PaleoValley.com Grass-fed Beef Sticks
- A small piece of fruit and a handful of nuts
- Veggies with guacamole
- Organic lunch meat spread with quality mayo or guacamole, rolled up alone or in a romaine lettuce leaf
- Olives like Lindsay Naturals, with a small piece of fruit or veggies
- Apple slices and sunbutter or almond butter
- Veggies dipped in tuna salad or egg salad
- Leftovers: A bowl of chili, a piece of chicken, or soup

Black Olive Tapenade

Mix in a food processor and serve with veggies

- 1 cup Kalamata olives
- 2-3 Tbsp olive oil

- 1 clove garlic
- 1 Tbsp fresh lemon juice
- 1/4 tsp black pepper
- 1/4 tsp dried thyme
- 2 tsp fresh parsley
- 1/2 tsp dried basil

Kale Chips

- 1 bunch kale, washed
- 1 tablespoon olive oil or avocado oil
- 1 teaspoon Real Salt or other seasoning like garlic salt

1. Preheat an oven to 350 degrees F.

2. Line a cookie sheet with parchment paper.

3. With a knife or kitchen shears, carefully remove the leaves from the thick stems and tear into large pieces.

4. Thoroughly air dry kale before using or dry in a salad spinner.

5. In a bowl, mix the kale with olive or avocado oil.

6. Season with salt or optional herbs of choice.

7. Bake until the edges brown but are not burnt, 10 to 15 minutes.

8. Watch the leaves carefully in the last minutes of cooking time or they will burn.

9. Kale chips melt in your mouth. Eat them hot!

These recipes give you an easy way to plan your first few meals and snacks. Take the time to look through my Real Food Recipe Book. With more than 60 recipes, this book will help you enjoy getting back in the kitchen to quickly prepare delicious meals and snacks. You will find the recipe book and a menu plan when you join my Facebook group, Whole Healthy Journey.

CHAPTER 21

PHASE 2

REINTRODUCTION. HOW TO REINTRODUCE FOODS AFTER THE 30-DAY ELIMINATION DIET

Congratulations for sticking with the 30-day elimination diet!

If you didn't quite get on board yet, let me encourage you to stick with the elimination diet plan for a full 30 days. Four weeks is a small price to pay for the information that the elimination diet reveals, and the bonus is that you will look and feel so much better.

Read these comments from others who have completed the elimination diet and filled out a survey. As I said before, everyone who follows the Reclaim Diet plan is happy they committed to the plan and they love how their bodies responded to real food (I did not add all those exclamation marks—the folks were all so excited with their results).

- *If anyone would have told me that I would feel this good, I wouldn't have believed it.*
- *Two months of headaches completely GONE!*
- *I've lost 9 pounds, feel less bloated, and sleep better.*
- *I used to get so bloated, had heartburn, felt tired with no energy. I feel SO much better now!!! All of these things are gone!! I used to live on sweets. Now, it isn't even an option in my mind. The*

good thing is I DON'T even crave anything sweet!! I used to never eat any vegetables. I am now eating asparagus, broccoli, sweet potato and carrots. This is a big change for me, but a GREAT change!!!

- *Increased energy!*
- *It is so worth it. You can feel so much better than you do now. You won't miss what you think you can't live without.*
- *Down 10+ pounds. Digestion is definitely better, no bloating or gas pain.*
- *I had more energy, my senses were heightened, my mood was very steady. I did crave a sweet thing from time to time, but I don't miss the refined sugar.*
- *I lost 15 pounds. Lost 2" on my waist. Energy has improved. I used to take medicine daily for acid reflux, and now don't need to. Sleeping much better.*
- *I felt much healthier, could think clearer, my skin was healthier, overall I felt great!*
- *I definitely felt healthier—more energetic—and my focus was on wholesome foods instead of junk. My cravings for sugar were practically non-existent.*
- *Lost 10 pounds, skin clearer and softer, energy level higher, mind clearer, digestion good.*

Are you ready to experience your own results? Your story is waiting to be written! Once you finish Phase 1, the elimination diet, you are ready for Phase 2.

The reintroduction period is the second phase of the Reclaim Diet. You will reintroduce foods one at a time, as I recommend below. One new food is added every three days to allow for delayed food reactions, which may take up to 72 hours to manifest.

Now that your immune system has had 30 days to calm down and heal, you will add one food to provoke your immune system. If your body reacts with any symptoms within one to three days, stop eating the food, you have your answer. That food is not for you, for now. Your symptoms indicate that the food you are testing is triggering a reaction. Log everything in your food journal.

You may want to seek the advice of a nutritionist or health practitioner that understands food sensitivities and how to heal the gut.

How to reintroduce foods

- Reintroduce one new food and consume it three times a day for three days unless you experience any symptoms.

- Reintroduce foods in the order suggested below.

- While gluten, soy and corn are tested by eating one food for three days, dairy is a little bit different. You may be sensitive to milk sugar (lactose) and/or milk protein (whey and casein). Begin reintroducing dairy by testing hard cheese which has very little lactose and whey. Testing goat's milk cheddar is best (if you can find it) because goat's milk has a different type of casein, A2, than casein typically found in cow's milk,

A1. A1 casein causes more inflammatory reactions than A2 casein.

- Observe any unusual reactions that may occur over the three-day period.

- Any unusual symptoms should be assumed to be a reaction to the food being tested.

- Record the date and food tested and note all reactions and symptoms. Examples of symptoms to watch for are listed below.

- If you have any reaction or symptoms, it is advised to stop eating the food being tested. Stop the reintroduction of new foods for a few days to allow the symptoms to go away before testing another food.

- Keep any food that causes reactions and symptoms out of your diet for a few months while you let your body heal. Seek advice from a health practitioner who is well-versed in food sensitivities.

Here is the recommended testing order, after the 30-day elimination diet. Follow the general reintroduction guidelines above.

- *Gluten.* First, test gluten by eating some whole wheat pasta with meals.
- *Dairy.* Test dairy initially by eating hard cheese. If you can

find goat's milk cheddar, that is the best place to start, due to the issue of A1 and A2 casein discussed above. If you do not observe any symptoms from eating goat's milk cheddar cheese, then try cow's milk cheddar cheese. If you experience no symptoms, then try a soft cheese followed by plain, organic, full-fat yogurt. If you do not tolerate hard cheese, then stop testing dairy because you will also react to the other forms. I do not recommend drinking pasteurized and homogenized milk from conventionally raised animals.

- *Corn.* Purchase a bag of organic frozen corn and eat it with meals.

- *Soy.* Purchase a bag of organic frozen edamame and eat it with meals. If soy does not trigger a reaction, it is fine to eat some organic fermented soy (miso, tempeh, natto, tamari sauce), but I do not recommend adding back soy and soybean oil, as I discussed earlier in Chapter 13.

- *Peanuts.* Eat plain or salted, dry-roasted peanuts a few times a day. I do not recommend adding back peanuts, as I discussed earlier in Chapter 13.

There is no need to test processed food, preservatives and artificial ingredients as those are not recommended and known to cause reactions. Food dyes and preservatives have been shown to increase hyperactivity in kids. Hidden MSG in food can trigger migraines and is very difficult to identify from an ingredients label on a package of processed food.

Symptoms to watch for during Phase 2

Watch for any new symptom that pops up, either immediately or within three days of eating a new food. This includes headaches, rashes, itchy skin, congestion, an increased heart rate/pulse, ringing in the ears, a feeling of water in the ears, joint or muscle aches and pains, feeling unwell, unusually tired, itching in the mouth, stomach aches, mucous in the throat, diarrhea or constipation, or sleep disturbances. Once you experience any symptom, stop eating the new food. If you are unsure, stop eating the food for a week and try to reintroduce it once again. As you test foods, even if they do not cause any symptoms, do not add the food back until you have completed Phase 2.

Join our online community, Whole Healthy Journey

I mentioned earlier that I host a free private Facebook group, Whole Healthy Journey. There are many resources there that clearly outline the elimination diet, and you will find educational videos that I have recorded, as well as a recipe book to give you many delicious, simple recipes. This is a community of wonderful folks who would love to encourage you on your journey. For access to the group, message me on Facebook if you cannot find the group.

CHAPTER 22

PHASE 3

INDIVIDUALIZATION. CUSTOMIZING YOUR OWN REAL FOOD PLAN

As you have followed the plan for the past few weeks, you have been eating an anti-inflammatory, healing, real food diet. You completed the 30-day elimination diet and then reintroduced certain foods to see how your body responds. Now you are ready to take the information you learned and continue on to the next phase of the Reclaim Diet, individualization—customizing the plan for you as an individual.

Moving forward, you now know the foods to avoid. Perhaps when you added dairy foods during Phase 2 you experienced congestion or digestive issues. Conventional dairy should be avoided by those who have sinus issues, asthma, allergies, and digestive issues. Dairy is not a food recommended for people with leaky gut, autoimmune conditions or gluten sensitivity. People who react to gluten tend to also react to dairy. Maybe you felt fine when you tested goat's milk cheese but did not tolerate cow's milk cheese. That indicates that you tolerate the casein (A2) found in goat's milk and can probably add that type of cheese back.

Review Chapter 13 before adding dairy, soy, grain and legumes back into your regular diet—we talked about many health issues with these foods, a reality of our modern world that many traditional cultures never had to consider.

I do not recommend adding back processed food, most legumes and grains. Organic quinoa and white rice can be eaten occasionally, if desired, keeping the serving size to 1/2 cup eaten with a meal containing protein, fat and vegetables. Organic lentils, if properly prepared by soaking and cooking (as we discussed in Chapter 13), can also be eaten occasionally.

Continue to enjoy eating three meals and include quality animal protein, healthy fat and vegetables. Explore new recipes and recipe books that focus on eating a whole-food diet. The internet is a great resource for finding recipes. If you use the search terms "paleo" or "AIP" you are more likely to find recipes that eliminate grains, dairy, soy and peanuts.

CHAPTER 23

PHASE 4

LIFESTYLE. MOVING FORWARD ON YOUR HEALTH JOURNEY

My first elimination diet was life-changing for me. I left the standard American diet and a world of fast-food, quickie processed meals, pudding cups, ice cream, cookies, soda and chips overnight. I was desperate for answers and needed healing from chronic hives. I knew very little about conditions that I was experiencing, like panic attacks, hives and Hashimoto's thyroiditis, but I knew that conventional medicine failed me by only offering prescription medications.

The elimination diet worked, slowly my skin cleared, and after more than 2 years, I was hive-free. I felt stuck in the elimination diet phase, afraid to deviate from what was working, I ate the same thing for breakfast for more than one year, eggs, mushrooms and asparagus. This was not a good idea, and now I know that we need to rotate food, and not eat any one food every single day, or risk developing a new food sensitivity. It is called dietary diversity; don't eat the same thing everyday.

As I help others begin the Reclaim Diet, I sometimes see myself in them. Usually, after the 30-day elimination diet, people feel so good, they do not want to do Phase 2 and test foods.

That is an option, but you may need to go through Phase 2 in order to have a clear understanding of how your body reacts to certain foods.

You can learn from my mistakes. After my first elimination diet, I continued on, feeling great. I felt so great, I decided that I could probably eat some processed food. It was a slippery slope, and all the addictive qualities of processed food drew me back in quickly. I was eating fast food, justifying in my mind that I was too busy working to stop and prepare lunch. I was buying Girl Scout cookies, ostensibly to help the scouts out, but eating the whole box by myself. I was treating the elimination diet like a prescription drug—using it to get the results I needed, then going back to the standard American diet.

It took another health scare or two to get my attention. I lost my voice for a few months—a vocal cord suddenly became paralyzed and this kept me in the medical system for CT scans, MRIs, ultrasounds, and mammograms. With all that poking and prodding, doctors found nothing wrong with my vocal cord but on their "fishing expedition" they found what they thought was breast cancer and recommended surgery that week! The surgeon told me, "It is an early cancer. If left alone, it is very, very, very likely to turn into a full blown cancer." He gave me two options, lumpectomy or mastectomy. I made an appointment for later that week for a lumpectomy to remove an egg-sized piece of tissue.

By the grace of God, I requested a copy of the pathology report and googled my diagnosis that evening. I was startled to read that surgery was not recommended and I sought a second opinion. I was led to the right physician who confirmed that I did not have breast cancer and I did not have a precancerous lesion. There was no reason for surgery. This horrible series of events lasted over four months, but I am grateful because it put a fire in my belly and a new determination to live the healthiest life possible so that I avoid being sucked into the SICKcare system ever again. The experience ramped up my enthusiasm for natural medicine and led me to pursue a Master's degree in holistic nutrition education.

When you complete Phase 1, 2 and 3 of the Reclaim Diet, you are at a crossroads. There is a decision to make. Will you continue on with the real food eating plan, and stay off processed foods and the high-carb standard American diet? I encourage you to steer clear of the slippery slope with processed food, factory-farmed dairy, refined grains and inflammatory oils.

We want to make this a lifestyle and not a short-term diet. This plan is a healthy human diet that will serve you well. Even though you may be in the beginning stages, now is a good time to think about what I asked you earlier:

Are you or were you:

- Sick or suffering
- Fat or frustrated

- Tired or wired
- Moody or medicated
- Despondent or depressed
- Anxious or agitated
- Pained and inflamed
- Sugar or grain-addicted

By following the Reclaim Diet, you have seen many positive changes in a short amount of time. Now, you will continue to heal your body and enjoy vibrant health.

This is the beginning of your real food journey, and now let's talk about tips for making it a lifestyle that you love.

You are an individual and now you know how your body is responding to certain foods. Real food works for everyone because this is a nutrient-rich way of eating that eliminates refined carbohydrates and processed foods. We have removed the sugars, dyes, chemicals, preservatives, and refined grains that are detrimental to digestive health and lead to inflammation. Avoiding conventionally-grown grains and legumes, and choosing organic produce, quality animal foods and healthy fats, dramatically reduced your intake of the herbicide, Roundup.

In the beginning stages, people tend to focus on foods they need to avoid, but transition to thinking about foods to enjoy. I do not recommend obsessing over calories, logging every morsel, and tracking your macros.

I do recommend eating PFV at meals, keeping basic guidelines in mind for each meal:

- Moderate animal protein. Portion size, about 3 or 4 ounces (20 to 30 grams).
- Healthy fat. One tablespoon of added fat, about 10 to 12 grams.
- Vegetables. Aim for two to three servings per meal and six to nine servings per day.
- Fruit. Zero to three servings of whole fruit per day, eaten at the end of a meal or with healthy fat and protein.
- Nuts. Limit nuts to one or two servings, 1/4 cup per serving.
- Seeds. Limit to a few tablespoons per day.

Adhering to the Reclaim Diet principles will become easier over time. You will see positive changes as your body heals and your comfort level with the eating plan will increase. This is the phase to experiment and try new recipes. Searching the internet using the term "paleo" or "AIP" will return many fabulous grain-free, dairy-free, real food recipes.

Pay attention to the ingredients used in recipes, as some bloggers are promoting a remake of the standard American diet. I have seen recipes for wheat-free, sweet potato brownies, full of starchy real food carbs, that were 36 grams of carbohydrates per brownie. This turns into 9 teaspoons of sugar in your bloodstream. These brownies may have real food ingredients, but they will be detrimental to insulin levels and weight loss efforts.

Those with sugar addictions will overeat these treats. Always eat nutrient-rich foods at meals and allow about four hours between meals without snacking. Initially, most people will need one snack between meals as they adjust to a lower carbohydrate, higher fat intake. Eventually, you may choose to drop the snack and focus on eating only at three mealtimes. I recommend not eating after dinner until breakfast, a period of about 12 hours. Try it for a while to determine if it improves your sleep. This does not work for everyone, and some people really do have better results by including a healthy bedtime snack, at least in the first month or two.

In Part 2, I gave a few tips for improving sleep. One tip I gave was to have a bedtime snack because I know that there is a transition period when people first switch away from the standard American diet to low-carb, real food. Eventually, as your body heals and adjusts to burning fat for fuel instead of carbs from crackers, chips and sweet treats, you can again try to skip the bedtime snack and enjoy the health and weight loss benefits that come from not eating after dinner.

Intermittent fasting and restricted eating times

There are many proponents of fasting and restricting the window of time for eating. In the beginning, be careful if you choose to go longer than a 12-hour overnight fast, especially if you are a woman or already thin. Women will experience a different response in hormones, which may change their menstrual cycle, affect fertility and cause a decrease in libido. Women with a history of disordered eating do not need another excuse to restrict themselves and increase stress.

Get healthy and fit by nourishing your body with the Reclaim Diet.

For those who want to go beyond a 12-hour fast, once you are no longer eating refined foods, and happily enjoying PFVx3 meals and have dropped between-meal snacks, a longer fast may be an option you choose to try. Fasting overnight and through breakfast (16 hours) brings benefits for insulin levels. Insulin levels are low, your body burns stored glucose and eventually turns to burning stored fat for fuel. For more information on fasting, seek out real food experts like Jason Fung, MD, and Ted Naiman, MD.

Are too many healthy snacks keeping you from achieving the next level of health?

Debbie and her husband, in their 50s, were eating healthy food, but decided to experiment with how often they ate and love the results.

"One big change Craig and I have made this year, we don't allow ourselves to eat after 6 p.m. (sometimes there are exceptions, of course, but the majority of the time, no!) and then we don't have breakfast until at least 9 a.m. or 10 a.m. For 15 to 16 hours we have nothing but water. We eat three balanced, whole food meals a day between 9 a.m. and 6 p.m. We have noticed a "reset" in our bodies, all sugar and food cravings are gone and we are feeling fantastic." — Debbie Prather

What about cheat days or the 80:20 rule?

The 80:20 principle can apply for some individuals but I am not a fan of the concept. The idea of having a "cheat" day assumes that some food is bad, and you deserve a break from your real food way of eating to kick up your heels for a day of unrestricted eating.

It is important to go back to how you felt during Phase 1, and what you learned about how your body reacts to certain foods in Phase 2. Think about your health goals. Connect the dots in your mind on how you feel after consuming certain food. For me, I had to have a conversation with myself in the beginning of my real food journey. "That cake looks good, but I know if I eat it, I will start getting itchy hives, and have a stomach ache. That wheat flour and sugar will be really hard for my thyroid and can set my healing back for weeks."

Over time, the Reclaim Diet way of eating became my new lifestyle. I prefer to eat unprocessed food and have found recipes to make a low-carb, grain-free treat like a "keto mug cake" if I really want a little dessert that won't hurt. I know I can have a square of 70% or higher dark chocolate now and then. I want to feel great, look great, keep autoimmune conditions and inflammation low. I want to stop any unnecessary surges of insulin and glucose because I value my life.

If you discovered that you have a sensitivity to gluten, eating food with gluten will bring back old problems and inflammation. Even a bite of a donut can trigger your immune system. You will not feel well, and it isn't just for a day—it can last for days, weeks or months.

When eating at a restaurant, or attending a party with friends, learn how to ask questions about food before consuming it. At a restaurant, tell the server that you cannot have any gluten.

Order a burger without the bun and get a side salad instead of fries that are made in a shared fryer of soybean oil contaminated by the chicken nuggets.

Instead of a "cheat day" you might have a "treat meal" where you have a piece of gluten-free bread for Sunday brunch. Gluten-free bread has more refined ingredients and higher carbs than you would expect, so consider that it is a refined carb that may not support your goals for managing insulin, glucose and weight.

If you feel completely healthy, and do not appear to have any specific food sensitivities and you eat clean most of the time, there may be room for a treat meal or two in a social situation.

The health you desire begins in your mind first. Decide what you want. Decide what leeway you will allow or not allow. Choose to be well, choose to learn the truth, choose to lean in to the information that has been presented to you in this book. You are valuable and you deserve to look and feel your best.

CHAPTER 24

REAL FOOD STORIES — LET'S WRITE YOUR STORY

Throughout this book I have shared many stories with you showing how people have faced their health challenges by optimizing their nutrition.

Part 1 Success Stories

Melissa (Chapter 1) overcame extreme fatigue, pain, depression, and rosacea, and she lost 26 pounds.

Jim (Chapter 2) lost 45 pounds and dropped his blood sugar levels from over 400mg/dl to an average of 95 - 115mg/dl and was able to come off several medications.

Ann (Chapter 3) found that following this plan led to resolution of several chronic health conditions including daily headaches, eczema, hives, fibromyalgia, fatigue, brain fog and depression.

Stephanie (Chapter 4) lost 25 pounds and balanced her emotions and hormones. She is no longer moody and bloated. She is able to sleep and focus.

Heidi (Chapter 5) lost 30 pounds and rarely has cravings now. She is no longer groggy in the afternoon and has seen improvements in her skin and hair too.

Part 2 Success Stories

Kris (Chapter 6) turned several chronic health problems around, including fibromyalgia, rosacea, stress and heart palpitations. In five months, she lost 50 pounds without even thinking about calories.

A 14-year-old girl (Chapter 7) found that a gluten-free diet allowed her to experience complete regression of all symptoms that plagued her for years, including daily headaches, difficulty concentrating, difficulty sleeping, poor behavior at home and school, crying spells and apathy.

Cecelia (Chapter 8) lost 30 pounds, rid herself of panic attacks, hair loss, massive pain, numbness in her face, swelling in her neck and chronic inflammation.

Steve (Chapter 9) lost 30 pounds, improved his blood sugar levels and came off several prescription medications. His energy levels are higher throughout the day.

Brian (Chapter 10) lost 20 pounds and no longer needs a CPAP machine.

Part 3 Success Stories

Kathy (Chapter 11) no longer needed multiple medications for asthma, allergies, pain and swelling. She suffered for 10 years and lost her ability to enjoy life, until she changed her diet and got off processed food, gluten and dairy.

Melissa Foster (Chapter 12) lost 37 pounds and found that following my eating plan led to a tremendous reduction in inflammation, pain, vertigo and brain fog. Her husband lost 20 pounds and saw fantastic improvements in his blood sugar control for type 2 diabetes.

Tracie (Chapter 13) and her husband together lost 91 pounds. Following this plan allowed them to heal from chronic health conditions like acid reflux, heartburn, digestive complaints, lack of energy and rosacea. Tracie's husband no longer needed insulin to control his blood sugar levels.

It is time to write your story.

The choice is yours. Will you choose to follow the plan and do the elimination diet? It takes courage to begin and to be "all in" but it is worth it. You are worth it and you deserve to look and feel your best.

I challenge you to follow Phase 1 of the plan for 30 days and you will enjoy a level of health that you never thought possible.

If you have been feeling like your health is moving downhill and you need a solid plan for losing weight, boosting energy, and sleeping better—it is time to take action and reclaim your health. The information presented in this book is transformational. It led myself and many others to finally get the health breakthrough we wanted. You have the power to change your life and set a new course. The next step is yours. Let's go reclaim your health!

I would love to hear your story, so be sure to reach out to me via social media or email, Erin@GetBetterWellness.com and join our community on Facebook at **Whole Healthy Journey** so that we can stay in touch!

APPENDIX A

GROCERY SHOPPING GUIDE

Stocking your kitchen to prepare for your real food journey is an important step for success. Try to plan three to seven days at a time when shopping. Meat, fish and chicken can always go in the freezer if you find a bargain. Until you get a feel for how much fresh produce you will be eating, you may want to plan your menu and meals for three days and only buy what is on the plan.

In the beginning when you are just starting out, don't worry too much about organic foods if it is difficult for you to source. First, simply focus on eating nutritious real food. As you progress on your journey, you can begin to scout out better quality foods and sources for organic animal protein and produce. Visit EWG.org/foodnews and download "EWG's Shopper's Guide to Pesticides in Produce." Buying organic versions of the "Dirty 12" (strawberries, spinach, kale, nectarines, apples, grapes, peaches, cherries, pears, tomatoes, celery and potatoes) helps you skip toxic chemicals. Buying conventional versions of the "Clean 15" (avocados, onions, asparagus, cabbage, cauliflower, broccoli, mushrooms and others) helps your wallet.

Animal Protein

The majority of your food budget is spent on high quality animal protein.

When the budget allows, choose grass-fed or organic meats and free-range (pasture-raised) poultry to avoid residues from antibiotics and pesticides.

Beef, pork, lamb, venison, wild game, bison

- Beef, ground and all cuts such as roasts, ribs, steaks and tips
- Pork, bacon, ham and sausage, roasts, ribs, loin, chops or steaks
- Lamb
- Venison and other wild game
- Bison

Poultry and Eggs

- Chicken - whole or parts
- Turkey - whole or parts
- Duck - whole or parts
- Other birds such as quail, Cornish hens, goose, ostrich
- Organic, pasture-raised eggs are nutrient dense and an inexpensive protein option

Deli Meats - Organic when possible

- Cold cuts such as turkey, chicken, ham
- Pepperoni slices
- Salami
- Prosciutto

Seafood

- Fresh or frozen fish of any kind, wild caught is best
- Canned fish such as sardines, tuna and salmon, water or oil packed (ideally olive oil or avocado oil)
- Fresh or frozen shellfish such as shrimp, scallops or crab

Vegetables - go for variety, and choose colorful options

- Bell peppers
- Broccoli
- Cucumbers
- Cabbage
- Cauliflower
- Green Beans
- Asparagus
- Brussels sprouts
- Celery
- Tomato
- Mushrooms

- Lettuce: large leaves can act as the "bread" for sandwiches (all varieties except iceberg)
- Leafy green vegetables such as collard, spinach and kale
- Onions, leeks and garlic, for flavorful cooking
- Root vegetables: carrots, beets, turnips, parsnips, rutabaga, sweet potato, radish, Jerusalem artichoke, yam, cassava
- Sprouts for salads
- Squash - zucchini, yellow, spaghetti, butternut

Nuts and seeds - raw, dry roasted, or sprouted

- Nuts: coconut, almonds, hazelnuts, pecans, walnuts, macadamia, pistachios, pine nuts, Brazil nuts (1/4 c. serving, one to two times per day)
- Nut flours like coconut flour and almond flour
- Seeds: sunflower, pumpkin, flax, sesame seeds

Fruit (0 to 3 servings per day)

- Avocados
- Choose lower sugar fruits that are high in nutrition like berries, tangerine, kiwi, oranges, coconut, peaches, cantaloupe, apples, cherries, lemon, lime, olives, passion fruit and persimmon.
- Limit high-carb fruits: bananas (1/2 banana is a serving) and plantains (1/4 is a serving), watermelon (1-2 cups), pineapple (½ cup) papaya (½ cup), mango (½ cup)
- Dried fruit is not recommended. It is very sugary and often contaminated with mold.

Fats

- Organic butter, Kerrygold butter, Organic Valley
- Organic ghee
- Extra-virgin olive oil
- Avocado oil
- Macadamia nut oil
- Coconut oil, unrefined, raw
- Canned coconut milk (full fat)
- Mayonnaise (avocado oil or coconut oil, such as Chosen Foods)

Pantry Items (organic when possible)

- Tomato products, marinara sauce, sun-dried tomatoes in oil
- Bubbies sauerkraut, dill pickles (refrigerated section of the produce department)
- Green chiles, roasted red peppers, chipotle peppers, mushrooms, artichoke hearts, hearts of palm
- Chicken, beef and vegetable stock, bone broth (gluten-free, organic)
- Nut and seed butters (natural, unsweetened)
- Ketchup (organic, limited use as it is high in sugar)
- Mustard (stone ground mustard, gluten-free)
- Raw apple cider vinegar, balsamic vinegar, wine vinegar
- Hot sauces (TABASCO®, Frank's® RedHot, sriracha)
- Most salsas (read ingredients)

- Coconut aminos, Coconut Secret (gluten-free, soy-free replacement for soy sauce)
- Mayonnaise (full fat, avocado- or coconut oil-based)
- Salad dressings, ideally homemade using olive or avocado oil
- Capers
- Horseradish (not horseradish sauces)
- Olives (look for olives in salt and water, like Lindsay Naturals)
- Beef sticks or jerky (PaleoValley.com, or Nicks-Sticks.com)
- Canned coconut milk, full fat like Natural Value or Native Forest
- Shredded coconut, unsweetened
- Coconut butter
- Bragg nutritional yeast
- Unrefined mineral salt (Redmond Real Salt˚ has 60+ trace minerals and no additives)

Cooking and Baking Ingredients

- Grass-fed collagen for smoothies (Vital Proteins Collagen Peptides)
- Sweet Leaf liquid stevia drops
- Raw cacao powder, organic
- Almond flour or other nut flours: keep these in freezer
- Pepper, Real Salt, cinnamon, garlic powder, chili powder, cayenne, oregano, basil, thyme, cumin, onion powder (organic)
- Raw honey
- Unrefined maple syrup

APPENDIX B

RESOURCES

Food

Refer to Appendix A, Grocery Shopping Guide.

Amazon Store for recommendations - Get Better Wellness

Amazon.com/shop/GetBetterWellness

- Healthy Fats and Oils
- Protein Sources
- MCT - Coconut Oil - Bulletproof Supplements
- Pantry
- Healthy Snacking
- Herbs, Tea, Spices
- Coffee
- Sprouting and Microgreens
- Silicone in the Kitchen
- Food Storage
- Cookware, Bakeware, Stoneware
- Kitchen Gadgets
- Detox and Sauna
- Books for Health and Wellness

Basic supplements that most people need

GetBetterWellness.com/supplements/

Magnesium Glycinate Complex, Klaire Labs

Vitamin D3 with K2

- D3 5,000 + K, Metagenics
- Vitamin D3 with K2 Liquid, Ortho Molecular

Omega-3s

- OmegaGize, Young Living
- Cod Liver Oil Lemon, Carlson

Digestive Enzymes

- EssentialZymes-4, Young Living

Probiotic

- Life 9, Young Living
- Complete Probiotics 70 Billion CFU, Mercola

Antioxidants

- NingXia Red, Young Living

Access Young Living supplements

- YoungLiving.com
- Save 24% by choosing a membership kit, enter 1277046 as enroller/sponsor to get a $25 resource package from me.

Access other supplements listed above

- https://wellevate.me/jacqueline-erin-chamerlik
- Save 15% when you register for a free account using the link above

Blue light protection glasses, SwannickSleep.com

CBD Tincture

Learn how to choose quality CBD and how to use CBD.

Educational video on my YouTube Channel, Erin Chamerlik.

GetBetterWellness.com/cbd101/

Epsom salts, unscented, Epsoak or Dr Teal's

Essential oils, Young Living

YoungLiving.com

Get a Premium Starter Kit and I will send you a $25 resource package (just enter 1277046 as enroller/sponsor at YoungLiving.com)

Wine

The best wine will be chemical-free, dry-farmed, grown organically or biodynamically farmed. See my blog post to learn how to avoid the 75 additives commonly added to most wine. I also help you learn how to find clean, low-carb wine that has been grown and fermented traditionally without the use of chemicals and toxins. GetBetterWellness.com/wine/

Appendix C

References

1.   Eisenberg, D. *Doctors need more nutrition education.* Harvard T.H. Chan School of Public Health News. hsph.harvard.edu

2.   Schwartz LM, Woloshin S. Medical Marketing in the United States, 1997-2016. *JAMA.* 2019;321(1):80–96. doi:10.1001/jama.2018.19320

3.   de Beer JC, Liebenberg L. Does cancer risk increase with HbA1c, independent of diabetes? Br J Cancer. 2014 Apr 29;110(9):2361-8. doi: 10.1038/bjc.2014.150. Epub 2014 Mar 27. PubMed PMID: 24675382; PubMed Central PMCID: PMC4007234.

4.   Alvheim AR, Malde MK, Osei-Hyiaman D, Lin YH, Pawlosky RJ, Madsen L, Kristiansen K, Frøyland L, Hibbeln JR. Dietary linoleic acid elevates endogenous 2-AG and anandamide and induces obesity. Obesity (Silver Spring). 2012 Oct;20(10):1984-94. doi: 10.1038/oby.2012.38. Epub 2012 Feb 15. PubMed PMID: 22334255; PubMed Central PMCID: PMC3458187.

5.   Blasbalg TL, Hibbeln JR, Ramsden CE, Majchrzak SF, Rawlings RR. Changes in consumption of omega-3 and omega-6 fatty acids in the United States during the 20th century. Am J Clin Nutr. 2011 May;93(5):950-62. doi: 10.3945/ajcn.110.006643. Epub 2011 Mar 2. PubMed PMID: 21367944; PubMed Central PMCID: PMC3076650.

6.   Ochsner Clinic and Alton Ochsner Medical Foundation. Syndrome X: A Short History. Gerald M. Reaven, MD
http://www.ochsnerjournal.org/content/ochjnl/3/3/124.full.pdf

7.   Thomas DD, Corkey BE, Istfan NW, Apovian CM. Hyperinsulinemia: An Early Indicator of Metabolic Dysfunction. J Endocr Soc. 2019 Sep 1;3(9):1727-1747. doi: 10.1210/js.2019-00065. eCollection 2019 Sep 1. Review. PubMed PMID: 31528832; PubMed Central PMCID: PMC6735759.

8.   Fung, J., Berger, A. Hyperinsulinemia and Insulin Resistance: Scope of the Problem. Journal of Insulin Resistance, Vol 1, No 1 (2016).

9.   Hu FB, Stampfer MJ, Rimm EB, Manson JE, Ascherio A, Colditz GA, Rosner BA, Spiegelman D, Speizer FE, Sacks FM, Hennekens CH, Willett WC. A prospective study of egg consumption and risk of cardiovascular disease in men and women. JAMA. 1999 Apr 21;281(15):1387-94. doi: 10.1001/jama.281.15.1387. PubMed PMID: 10217054.

10.   Zhong VW, Van Horn L, Cornelis MC, Wilkins JT, Ning H, Carnethon MR, Greenland P, Mentz RJ, Tucker KL, Zhao L, Norwood AF, Lloyd-Jones DM, Allen NB. Associations of Dietary Cholesterol or Egg Consumption With Incident Cardiovascular Disease and Mortality. JAMA. 2019 Mar 19;321(11):1081-1095. doi: 10.1001/jama.2019.1572. PubMed PMID: 30874756; PubMed Central PMCID: PMC6439941.

11.   Oz, Mehmet. (2019, April 4). The truth about eggs and heart health. *NewsMax Health*. Retrieved from NewsMax.com.

12.   Scher, B. (2019, December 31). Diet Doctor Podcast #36 - Dr. Eric Westman. *Diet Doctor*. Retrieved from DietDoctor.com

13. Johnston CS, Kim CM, Buller AJ. Vinegar improves insulin sensitivity to a high-carbohydrate meal in subjects with insulin resistance or type 2 diabetes. Diabetes Care. 2004 Jan;27(1):281-2. doi: 10.2337/diacare.27.1.281. PubMed PMID: 14694010.

14. Iman M. Effect of Apple Cider Vinegar on Blood Glucose Level in Diabetic Mice. Journal of pharmaceutical sciences. 2015 March; 20(4):163-168.

15. Claesson AL, Holm G, Ernersson A, Lindström T, Nystrom FH. Two weeks of overfeeding with candy, but not peanuts, increases insulin levels and body weight. Scand J Clin Lab Invest. 2009;69(5):598-605. doi: 10.1080/00365510902912754. PubMed PMID: 19396658.

16. Ebbeling, C.B. et al. Effects of Dietary Composition on Energy Expenditure During Weight-Loss Maintenance. *JAMA*, June 27, 2012 DOI: 10.1001/jama.2012.6607

17. Volek J, Sharman M, Gómez A, Judelson D, Rubin M, Watson G, Sokmen B, Silvestre R, French D, Kraemer W. Comparison of energy-restricted very low-carbohydrate and low-fat diets on weight loss and body composition in overweight men and women. Nutr Metab (Lond). 2004 Nov 8;1(1):13. doi: 10.1186/1743-7075-1-13. PubMed PMID: 15533250; PubMed Central PMCID: PMC538279.

18. Lionetti E, Leonardi S, Franzonello C, Mancardi M, Ruggieri M, Catassi C. Gluten Psychosis: Confirmation of a New Clinical Entity. Nutrients. 2015 Jul 8;7(7):5532-9. doi: 10.3390/nu7075235. PubMed PMID: 26184290; PubMed Central PMCID: PMC4517012.

19.   Fasano A. Surprises from celiac disease. Sci Am. 2009 Aug;301(2):54-61. doi: 10.1038/scientificamerican0809-54. PubMed PMID: 19634568.

20.   University of Oslo. "Being overweight causes hazardous inflammations." ScienceDaily. ScienceDaily, 25 August 2014. www.sciencedaily.com/releases/2014/08/140825084836.htm

21.   Alcohol and the Immune System. 10th Special Report to the U.S. Congress on Alcohol and Health. Medical Consequences, Chapter 4. https://pubs.niaaa.nih.gov/publications/10report/intro.pdf

22.   Hess J, Bednarz D, Bae J, Pierce J. Petroleum and health care: evaluating and managing health care's vulnerability to petroleum supply shifts. Am J Public Health. 2011 Sep;101(9):1568-79. doi: 10.2105/AJPH.2011.300233. Epub 2011 Jul 21. PubMed PMID: 21778473; PubMed Central PMCID: PMC3154246.

23.   Mullington JM, Simpson NS, Meier-Ewert HK, Haack M. Sleep loss and inflammation. Best Pract Res Clin Endocrinol Metab. 2010 Oct;24(5):775-84. doi: 10.1016/j.beem.2010.08.014. Review. PubMed PMID: 21112025; PubMed Central PMCID: PMC3548567.

24.   Choi Y, Chang Y, Ryu S, Cho J, Rampal S, Zhang Y, Ahn J, Lima JA, Shin H, Guallar E. Coffee consumption and coronary artery calcium in young and middle-aged asymptomatic adults. Heart. 2015 May;101(9):686-91. doi: 10.1136/heartjnl-2014-306663. Epub 2015 Mar 2. PubMed PMID: 25732752.

25.   Palsdottir, H. (2016, August 12). Is coffee good for your brain? Retrieved from healthline.com on September 12, 2019.

26.   Shield K, Soerjomataram I, Rehm J. Alcohol Use and Breast Cancer: A Critical Review. Alcohol clin Exp Res. 2016 Jun;40(6):1166-81. doi: 10.1111/acer.13071.

27.   Li Y, Li S, Zhou Y, et al. Melatonin for the prevention and treatment of cancer. Oncotarget. 2017;8(24):39896–39921. doi:10.18632/oncotarget.16379

28.   Donga E, van Dijk M, van Dijk JG, Biermasz NR, Lammers GJ, van Kralingen KW, Corssmit EP, Romijn JA. A single night of partial sleep deprivation induces insulin resistance in multiple metabolic pathways in healthy subjects. J Clin Endocrinol Metab. 2010 Jun;95(6):2963-8. doi: 10.1210/jc.2009-2430. Epub 2010 Apr 6. PubMed PMID: 20371664.

29.   Watson NF, Badr MS, Belenky G, et al. Recommended Amount of Sleep for a Healthy Adult: A Joint Consensus Statement of the American Academy of Sleep Medicine and Sleep Research Society. *Sleep.* 2015;38(6):843–844. Published 2015 Jun 1. doi:10.5665/sleep.4716

30.   Nedeltcheva AV, Kilkus JM, Imperial J, Schoeller DA, Penev PD. Insufficient sleep undermines dietary efforts to reduce adiposity. Ann Intern Med. 2010 Oct 5;153(7):435-41. doi: 10.7326/0003-4819-153-7-201010050-00006. PubMed PMID: 20921542; PubMed Central PMCID: PMC2951287.

31.   Emet M, Ozcan H, Ozel L, Yayla M, Halici Z, Hacimuftuoglu A. A Review of Melatonin, Its Receptors and Drugs. Eurasian J Med. 2016 Jun;48(2):135-41. doi: 10.5152/eurasianjmed.2015.0267. Review. PubMed PMID: 27551178; PubMed Central PMCID: PMC4970552.

32.   Pilcher JJ, Huffcutt AI. Effects of sleep deprivation on performance: a meta-analysis. Sleep. 1996 May;19(4):318-26. doi: 10.1093/sleep/19.4.318. PubMed PMID: 8776790.

33.   Gramlich LM, Olstad DL, Nasser R, Goonewardene L, Raman M, Innis S, Wicklum S, Duerksen D, Rashid M, Heyland D, Armstrong D, Roy C. Medical students' perceptions of nutrition education in Canadian universities. Appl Physiol Nutr Metab. 2010 Jun;35(3):336-43. doi: 10.1139/H10-016. PubMed PMID: 20555378.

34.   Collaborators. Health effects of dietary risks in 195 countries, 1990-2017: a systematic analysis for the Global Burden of Disease Study 2017. Lancet. 2019 May 11;393(10184):1958-1972. doi: 10.1016/S0140-6736(19)30041-8. Epub 2019 Apr 4. PubMed PMID: 30954305.

35.   Wolf DM, Segawa M, Kondadi AK. Individual cristae within the same mitochondrion display different membrane potentials and are functionally independent. EMBO J. 2019 Oct 14. doi: 10.15252/embj.2018101056.

36.   Xiao M, Ya L, Sha L. Dietary Sources and Bioactivities of Melatonin. Nutrients. 2017 Apr; 9(4): 367. doi: 10.3390/nu9040367

37.   Banskota S, Ghia JE, Khan WI. Serotonin in the gut: Blessing or a curse. Biochimie. 2019 Jun;161:56-64. doi: 10.1016/j.biochi.2018.06.008. Epub 2018 Jun 14. Review. PubMed PMID: 29909048.

38.   Spreadbury I. Comparison with ancestral diets suggests dense acellular carbohydrates promote an inflammatory microbiota, and may be the primary dietary cause of leptin resistance and obesity. *Diabetes Metab Syndr Obes.* 2012;5:175–189. doi:10.2147/DMSO.S33473

39.   Volek JS, Phinney SD, Forsythe CE, Quann EE, Wood RJ, Puglisi MJ, Kraemer WJ, Bibus DM, Fernandez ML, Feinman RD. Carbohydrate restriction has a more favorable impact on the metabolic syndrome than a low fat diet._Lipids. 2009 Apr;44(4):297-309. doi: 10.1007/s11745-008-3274-2. Epub 2008 Dec 12. PubMed PMID: 19082851.

40.   Vasconcelos IM, Oliveira JT. Antinutritional properties of plant lectins._Toxicon. 2004 Sep 15;44(4):385-403. doi: 10.1016/j.toxicon.2004.05.005. Review. PubMed PMID: 15302522.

41.   Noonan SC, Savage GP. Oxalate content of foods and its effect on humans._Asia Pac J Clin Nutr. 1999 Mar;8(1):64-74. PubMed PMID: 24393738.

42.   Daniel, K. T. (2005). The Whole Soy Story. Washington D.C.: New Trends Publishing.

43.   Irvine, C. H., Fitzpatrick, M. G., Alexander, S. L., (1998). The Potential Adverse Effects of Soybean Phytoestrogens in Infant Feeding New Zealand Medical Journal 1995 May 24:318

44.   Wu F, Stacy SL, Kensler TW. Global risk assessment of aflatoxins in maize and peanuts: are regulatory standards adequately protective?. Toxicol Sci. 2013 Sep;135(1):251-9. doi: 10.1093/toxsci/kft132. Epub 2013 Jun 12. PubMed PMID: 23761295; PubMed Central PMCID: PMC3748761.

45.   Gillam, C. "Monsanto Roundup Trial Tracker." *U.S. Right to Know. 13 Nov. 2019.* Web access date 22 Nov. 2019.

46. Temkin, A. "Glyphosate Contamination in Food Goes Far Beyond Oat Products." EWG.org Web access date 23 Nov. 2019.

47. Seneff S, Samsel A. Glyphosate, pathways to modern diseases II: Celiac sprue and gluten intolerance. Review article Interdiscip Toxicol. 2013 Dec; 6(4): 159–184.

48. ResponsibleTechnology.org "Glyphosate Testing Results." Web access date 23 Nov. 2019.

49. Park YW, Zhu S, Palaniappan L, Heshka S, Carnethon MR, Heymsfield SB. The metabolic syndrome: prevalence and associated risk factor findings in the US population from the Third National Health and Nutrition Examination Survey, 1988-1994. Arch Intern Med. 2003 Feb 24;163(4):427-36. doi: 10.1001/archinte.163.4.427. PubMed PMID: 12588201; PubMed Central PMCID: PMC3146257.

50. Kerr JR. Milk and mortality: raw versus pasteurised milk. BMJ. 2014 Nov 26;349:g6993. doi: 10.1136/bmj.g6993. PubMed PMID: 25427886.

51. Kresser, C. Why Eating Meat is Good for You. Access 2020 Jan 11. https://chriskresser.com/why-eating-meat-is-good-for-you/

52. Cofnas N. Is vegetarianism healthy for children?. Crit Rev Food Sci Nutr.2019;59(13):2052-2060. doi: 10.1080/10408398.2018.1437024. Epub 2018 Feb 23. Review. PubMed PMID: 29405739.

53. Gorvett, Z. (2020, January 27). How a vegan diet could affect your intelligence. BBC Future. Retrieved from BBC.com

54.   Van der Zee, B. (2017, October 4). Why factory farming is not just cruel — but also a threat to all life on the planet. The Guardian. Retrieved from TheGuardian.com

55.   Raynor HA, Goff MR, Poole SA, Chen G. Eating Frequency, Food Intake, and Weight: A Systematic Review of Human and Animal Experimental Studies. Front Nutr. 2015;2:38. Published 2015 Dec 18. doi:10.3389/fnut.2015.00038

56.   Murakami K, Livingstone MB. Eating Frequency Is Positively Associated with Overweight and Central Obesity in U.S. Adults. J Nutr. 2015 Dec;145(12):2715-24. doi: 10.3945/jn.115.219808. Epub 2015 Oct 14. PubMed PMID: 26468490.

57.   Badger, M. Pasture and Feed Affect Broiler Carcass Nutrition. 2015 Apr;
https://apppa.org/resources/Documents/Pasture%20and%20Feed%20Aff
ect%20Broiler%20Carcass%20Nutrition%20--Final%20-%20rev%204-
22-15.pdf

58.   Melgar MJ, Núñez R, García MÁ. Selenium intake from tuna in Galicia (Spain): Health risk assessment and protective role against exposure to mercury and inorganic arsenic. Sci Total Environ. 2019 Dec 1;694:133716. doi: 10.1016/j.scitotenv.2019.133716. Epub 2019 Aug 5. PubMed PMID: 31756789.

59.   Ahn JS, Kang KW, Kang WY, Lim HM, Cho S, Moon JD, Park WJ. Mercury poisoning in a fisherman working on a pelagic fishing vessel due to excessive tuna consumption. J Occup Health. 2018 Jan 25;60(1):89-93. doi: 10.1539/joh.16-0274-CS. Epub 2017 Nov 1. PubMed PMID: 29093364; PubMed Central PMCID: PMC5799106.

60.   Vital Choice. How much mercury is in your albacore compared to other tuna? Retrieved from VitalChoice.com

61.   Renaud S, de Lorgeril M. Wine, alcohol, platelets, and the French paradox for coronary heart disease. Lancet. 1992 Jun 20;339(8808):1523-6. doi: 10.1016/0140-6736(92)91277-f. PubMed PMID: 1351198.

62.   de Lorgeril M, Salen P, Paillard F, Laporte F, Boucher F, de Leiris J. Mediterranean diet and the French paradox: two distinct biogeographic concepts for one consolidated scientific theory on the role of nutrition in coronary heart disease. Cardiovasc Res. 2002 Jun;54(3):503-15. doi: 10.1016/s0008-6363(01)00545-4. Review. PubMed PMID: 12031696.

63.   Godfrey JR. A tour of school lunch: what we can learn from the French approach. Child Obes. 2012 Oct;8(5):491-5. doi: 10.1089/chi.2012.0085.lunc. PubMed PMID: 23061506.

64.   Coconut Research Center. http://www.coconutresearchcenter.org/?page_id=5173

65.   Freitas RDS, Campos MM. Protective Effects of Omega-3 Fatty Acids in Cancer-Related Complications. Nutrients. 2019 Apr 26;11(5). doi: 10.3390/nu11050945. Review. PubMed PMID: 31035457; PubMed Central PMCID: PMC6566772.

66.   Gammone MA, Riccioni G, Parrinello G, D'Orazio N. Omega-3 Polyunsaturated Fatty Acids: Benefits and Endpoints in Sport. Nutrients. 2018 Dec 27;11(1). doi: 10.3390/nu11010046. Review. PubMed PMID: 30591639; PubMed Central PMCID: PMC6357022.

67.   Lunn J., Theobald H. The health effects of dietary unsaturated fatty acids. Nutr. Bull. 2006;31:178–224. doi: 10.1111/j.1467-3010.2006.00571.x

68.   Ginty AT, Conklin SM. Short-term supplementation of acute long-chain omega-3 polyunsaturated fatty acids may alter depression status and decrease symptomology among young adults with depression: A preliminary randomized and placebo controlled trial. Psychiatry Res. 2015 Sep 30;229(1-2):485-9. doi: 10.1016/j.psychres.2015.05.072. Epub 2015 Jun 27. PubMed PMID: 26188642.

69.   Merle BM, Benlian P, Puche N, Bassols A, Delcourt C, Souied EH. Circulating omega-3 Fatty acids and neovascular age-related macular degeneration. Invest Ophthalmol Vis Sci. 2014 Mar 28;55(3):2010-9. doi: 10.1167/iovs.14-13916. PubMed PMID: 24557349.

70.   Peter S, Chopra S, Jacob JJ. A fish a day, keeps the cardiologist away! - A review of the effect of omega-3 fatty acids in the cardiovascular system. Indian J Endocrinol Metab. 2013 May;17(3):422-9. doi: 10.4103/2230-8210.111630. PubMed PMID: 23869297; PubMed Central PMCID: PMC3712371.

71.   McCusker MM, Grant-Kels JM. Healing fats of the skin: the structural and immunologic roles of the omega-6 and omega-3 fatty acids. Clin Dermatol. 2010 Jul-Aug;28(4):440-51. doi: 10.1016/j.clindermatol.2010.03.020. PubMed PMID: 20620762.

72.   Calder PC. Docosahexaenoic Acid. Ann Nutr Metab. 2016;69 Suppl 1:7-21. doi: 10.1159/000448262. Epub 2016 Nov 15. PubMed PMID: 27842299.

73.   Eades, M. A spoonful of sugar. Retrieved from
https://proteinpower.com/a-spoonful-of-sugar/

74.   White H, Venkatesh B. Clinical review: ketones and brain injury.
Crit Care. 2011 Apr 6;15(2):219. doi: 10.1186/cc10020. Review.
PubMed PMID: 21489321; PubMed Central PMCID: PMC3219306.

75.   Mercola, J. Fat for Fuel: Why Dietary Fat, Not Glucose, Is the
Preferred Body Fuel. 2012 Aug.
https://fitness.mercola.com/sites/fitness/archive/2012/08/10/fat-not-
glucose.aspx

76.   Sisson, M. A Metabolic Paradigm Shift, or Why Fat Is the Preferred
Fuel for Human Metabolism. Access 2019 Dec 20.
https://www.marksdailyapple.com/a-metabolic-paradigm-shift-fat-carbs-
human-body-metabolism/

77.   Page KA, Williamson A, Yu N, McNay EC, Dzuira J, McCrimmon
RJ, Sherwin RS. Medium-chain fatty acids improve cognitive function in
intensively treated type 1 diabetic patients and support in vitro synaptic
transmission during acute hypoglycemia. Diabetes. 2009
May;58(5):1237-44. doi: 10.2337/db08-1557. Epub 2009 Feb 17.
PubMed PMID: 19223595; PubMed Central PMCID: PMC2671041.

78.   Reger MA, Henderson ST, Hale C, Cholerton B, Baker LD,
Watson GS, Hyde K, Chapman D, Craft S. Effects of beta-
hydroxybutyrate on cognition in memory-impaired adults. Neurobiol
Aging. 2004 Mar;25(3):311-4. doi: 10.1016/S0197-4580(03)00087-3.
PubMed PMID: 15123336.

79.   Krikorian R, Shidler MD, Dangelo K, Couch SC, Benoit SC, Clegg DJ. Dietary ketosis enhances memory in mild cognitive impairment. Neurobiol Aging. 2012 Feb;33(2):425.e19-27. doi: 10.1016/j.neurobiolaging.2010.10.006. Epub 2010 Dec 3. PubMed PMID: 21130529; PubMed Central PMCID: PMC3116949.

80.   Paoli A, Rubini A, Volek JS, Grimaldi KA. Beyond weight loss: a review of the therapeutic uses of very-low-carbohydrate (ketogenic) diets. Eur J Clin Nutr. 2013 Aug;67(8):789-96. doi: 10.1038/ejcn.2013.116. Epub 2013 Jun 26. Review. PubMed PMID: 23801097; PubMed Central PMCID: PMC3826507.

81.   Samaha FF, Iqbal N, Seshadri P, Chicano KL, Daily DA, McGrory J, Williams T, Williams M, Gracely EJ, Stern L. A low-carbohydrate as compared with a low-fat diet in severe obesity. N Engl J Med. 2003 May 22;348(21):2074-81. doi: 10.1056/NEJMoa022637. PubMed PMID: 12761364.

82.   Sondike SB, Copperman N, Jacobson MS. Effects of a low-carbohydrate diet on weight loss and cardiovascular risk factor in overweight adolescents. J Pediatr. 2003 Mar;142(3):253-8. doi: 10.1067/mpd.2003.4. PubMed PMID: 12640371.

83.   Brehm BJ, Seeley RJ, Daniels SR, D'Alessio DA. A randomized trial comparing a very low carbohydrate diet and a calorie-restricted low fat diet on body weight and cardiovascular risk factors in healthy women. J Clin Endocrinol Metab. 2003 Apr;88(4):1617-23. doi: 10.1210/jc.2002-021480. PubMed PMID: 12679447.

84. Tay J, Brinkworth GD, Noakes M, Keogh J, Clifton PM. Metabolic effects of weight loss on a very-low-carbohydrate diet compared with an isocaloric high-carbohydrate diet in abdominally obese subjects. J Am Coll Cardiol. 2008 Jan 1;51(1):59-67. doi: 10.1016/j.jacc.2007.08.050. PubMed PMID: 18174038.

85. Volek JS, Phinney SD, Forsythe CE, Quann EE, Wood RJ, Puglisi MJ, Kraemer WJ, Bibus DM, Fernandez ML, Feinman RD. Carbohydrate restriction has a more favorable impact on the metabolic syndrome than a low fat diet. Lipids. 2009 Apr;44(4):297-309. doi: 10.1007/s11745-008-3274-2. Epub 2008 Dec 12. PubMed PMID: 19082851.

86. Gepner Y, Shelef I, Komy O, Cohen N, Schwarzfuchs D, Bril N, Rein M, Serfaty D, Kenigsbuch S, Zelicha H, Yaskolka Meir A, Tene L, Bilitzky A, Tsaban G, Chassidim Y, Sarusy B, Ceglarek U, Thiery J, Stumvoll M, Blüher M, Stampfer MJ, Rudich A, Shai I. The beneficial effects of Mediterranean diet over low-fat diet may be mediated by decreasing hepatic fat content. J Hepatol. 2019 Aug;71(2):379-388. doi: 10.1016/j.jhep.2019.04.013. Epub 2019 May 8. PubMed PMID: 31075323.

87. Aude YW, Agatston AS, Lopez-Jimenez F, Lieberman EH, Marie Almon, Hansen M, Rojas G, Lamas GA, Hennekens CH. The national cholesterol education program diet vs a diet lower in carbohydrates and higher in protein and monounsaturated fat: a randomized trial. Arch Intern Med. 2004 Oct 25;164(19):2141-6. doi: 10.1001/archinte.164.19.2141. PubMed PMID: 15505128.

88.   Yancy WS Jr, Olsen MK, Guyton JR, Bakst RP, Westman EC. A low-carbohydrate, ketogenic diet versus a low-fat diet to treat obesity and hyperlipidemia: a randomized, controlled trial. Ann Intern Med. 2004 May 18;140(10):769-77. doi: 10.7326/0003-4819-140-10-200405180-00006. PubMed PMID: 15148063.

89.   Volek J, Sharman M, Gómez A, et al. Comparison of energy-restricted very low-carbohydrate and low-fat diets on weight loss and body composition in overweight men and women. Nutr Metab (Lond). 2004;1(1):13. Published 2004 Nov 8. doi:10.1186/1743-7075-1-13

90.   Nickols-Richardson SM, Coleman MD, Volpe JJ, Hosig KW. Perceived hunger is lower and weight loss is greater in overweight premenopausal women consuming a low-carbohydrate/high-protein vs high-carbohydrate/low-fat diet. J Am Diet Assoc. 2005 Sep;105(9):1433-7. doi: 10.1016/j.jada.2005.06.025. PubMed PMID: 16129086.

91.   McClernon FJ, Yancy WS Jr, Eberstein JA, Atkins RC, Westman EC. The effects of a low-carbohydrate ketogenic diet and a low-fat diet on mood, hunger, and other self-reported symptoms. Obesity (Silver Spring). 2007 Jan;15(1):182-7. doi: 10.1038/oby.2007.516. PubMed PMID: 17228046.

92.   Ebbeling CB, Feldman HA, Klein GL, Wong JMW, Bielak L, Steltz SK, Luoto PK, Wolfe RR, Wong WW, Ludwig DS. Effects of a low carbohydrate diet on energy expenditure during weight loss maintenance: randomized trial. BMJ. 2018 Nov 14;363:k4583. doi: 10.1136/bmj.k4583. PubMed PMID: 30429127; PubMed Central PMCID: PMC6233655.

93.   Westman EC, Yancy WS Jr, Mavropoulos JC, Marquart M, McDuffie JR. The effect of a low-carbohydrate, ketogenic diet versus a low-glycemic index diet on glycemic control in type 2 diabetes mellitus. Nutr Metab (Lond). 2008;5:36. Published 2008 Dec 19. doi:10.1186/1743-7075-5-36